QUALITY ASSURANCE IN NURSING

QUALITY ASSURANCE IN NURSING

Concepts, Methods and Case Studies

Heather Marr
Hannie Giebing

Campion Press

British Library Cataloguing in Publication Data

Giebing, H.
Quality Assurance in Nursing
I. Title II. Marr, H.
610.7307

ISBN 1-873732-04-X

© 1994
Campion Press Limited,
384 Lanark Road,
Edinburgh EH13 0LX

Cover design:
Artisan Graphics, Edinburgh

Page make-up
Word Power, Berwickshire

Typeset in Optima 10pt

Printed and bound by
The Alden Press, Oxford.

Translated sections by
L.F.M. van Beeck

Preface

During the course of the past decade or so, the fundamental changes which have taken place in the planning and provision of health care have resulted in an increased awareness of the concept, methods and development of quality assurance activity for those delivering health care. In some instances it is an activity which has been entered into willingly and indeed enthusiastically; in others it has been forced upon us as an uncomfortable consequence of these changes.

With the introduction of General Management through the *Griffiths' Enquiry* (1984), the philosophy of administration through consensus was replaced by the principles of management. Griffiths made strong recommendations for improved quality of service, defined mainly in terms of consumers' needs within a commercial service model. On an international note the WHO agreement in *Targets for Health for All* (1985) proclaimed that, by 1990, "We should have built effective mechanisms for ensuring quality of patient care within our health-care systems."

The White Papers *Working for Patients* (1990), and *Caring for People* (1991), offered opportunities and challenges for, and demanded major change from everyone working in the National Health Service. *Working for Patients* placed audit, both professional and financial, among the arrangements necessary to secure value for money in the NHS and at the same time set out to give patients, wherever they live in the UK, better health care and a greater choice of services available. In addition, this White Paper stressed the importance of providing greater satisfaction and rewards for those working in the NHS who successfully respond to local needs and preferences.

No other discipline within health care has responded by rising to the new challenges more than nursing has, hence many of those managers now responsible for directing and co-ordinating multiprofessional quality assurance activity have come from a nursing background. It is now generally acknowledged that quality assurance is a necessary part of nursing practice and this aspect of the profession is increasingly being integrated into every nurse's role and remit, senior or junior.

"Quality" is not just a fashionable buzz word: it is a concern which goes to the heart of nursing and is doomed to fail if it cannot find its rightful place among the accepted, everyday tools of the clinical nurse. That at least is the strongly held view of many nurses in key positions who have looked at standard setting and its important contribution to quality assurance, and of the growing number of clinical nurses who are setting and monitoring standards in many varying specialties.

Quality assurance in nursing can be regarded as an essential part of a total quality assurance system in patient care. Seen in this context, it is therefore timely and indeed imperative that it is examined in more detail. A number of pressures are being exercised both externally (as described above) and internally on the development of quality assurance in nursing. Such influences have been categorised by Kitson and Giebing (1990) as professional, legal, social and political, and together they all contribute to an increased awareness of the need for quality assurance in health care and in nursing in particular.

Another notable influence which increases the necessity to concern ourselves with issues of quality is the growing workload as a result of the reduced length of hospital stay requiring constant, intensive or semi-intensive nursing care. The consequences of the shorter stay patients are also felt within community health care and the experience of nurses in the community is that the need for such care is growing rapidly. Other factors which highlight the importance of quality assurance are the reduction of working hours, the steady expansion in the field of technical developments and the growing empowerment of clients and patients, who are increasingly regarded as having an independent, active input into their own treatment and whose expectations regarding care are ever-increasing. This accumulation of factors raises the question of these pressures affecting the quality of nursing care, hence the growing demand in the nursing profession for methods of assuring and improving quality in the management and delivery of care.

The book is written in two parts. Part One is concerned with the concept of quality in general, that of quality in nursing in particular, and ways of improving and assuring quality. A considerable amount of attention is devoted to assessing and evaluating at departmental level or at a local level - that is, a unit-based or decentralised and practitioner-based approach. Thousands of nurses along with other professionals have gained experience with this method of quality assurance and improvement throughout a number of European countries. In the light of their experiences, there is a great deal of interest by professionals internationally, both in hospital and community. Learning outcomes and study activities are given throughout Part One and it is hoped that the inclusion of these will help the student to comprehend the subject matter more fully.

In Part Two practical examples of this method of quality improvement are described as they have emerged from practice in seven factual experiences. Although these are described as case studies, they cannot be regarded as model standards and criteria sets from which can be deduced a general set of rules: instead, they illustrate how groups can utilise this dynamic approach to evaluate nursing practice using standard setting and criteria formulation, and they give practical examples of how such an approach to quality can be usefully applied in the real world.

This publication seeks therefore to provide insight into quality improvement and quality assurance activities in nursing. The authors hope that the inclusion of the case studies will encourage other groups to participate in the practical application. It is intended primarily for students of nursing on Project 2000 diploma courses but will also have relevance for those studying in post-diploma education, nurses who work in clinical practice and nurses in management

Due to the lack of a genderless singular personal pronoun in the English language it is difficult to achieve political correctness in a book such as this with constant references to the nurse and the patient. For convenience the authors refer to the nurse throughout in the female gender. Patients and clients are referred to in the male gender. Where there is no distinction between patients and clients the term *patient* is used rather than *patient/client*.

Heather Marr, Hannie Giebing
May, 1994.

Acknowledgements

The authors would like to acknowledge and thank the following people who have kindly given permission to reproduce some of their work.
The Royal College of Nursing for their extensive work on Standards of Nursing Care.
Alison Kitson and Gill Harvey, Institute of Nursing, Oxford, for their work on the Dynamic Standard Setting System and the role of the facilitator.
Daphne Bellingham, Kirkcaldy Hospitals, NHS Trust Fife, for her work on the Standard on Pain Management (Figure 1.4.4)
The Directorate of Quality and Patient Services, Fife Health Board for the Named Nurse (Figure 1.2.4) on page 34, Philosophy of Nurse Management on page 125 and Management Standards figures on pages 127–134.
Geraldine Cunningham, Royal Brompton National Heart and Lung Hospital for Part 2 Chapter 1.
Chrissy Dunn, Royal Berkshire and Battle NHS Trust for Part 2 Chapter 2.
Lynebank Hospital, Fife Healthcare NHS Trust for their quality improvement activity described in Chapter 3.
Accident and Emergency Staff, Queen Margaret Hospital, NHS Trust, Fife for their quality improvement activity described in Part 2 Chapter 4.
Morag Hamil, Health Promotion Specialist, Fife, James Slaven, Anthea Lokko and Julie Gharabally, Fife Healthcare NHS Trust for the Patient Education Standard activity described in Part 2 Chapter 4.
Community Nursing Staff, Fife Healthcare NHS Trust for Part 2 Chapter 5 …and finally, family and friends for their patience and support during this never-ending-story!

Contents

PART TWO
CASE STUDIES - EXPERIENCES WITH LOCALLY ORGANISED METHODS

PART ONE
CONCEPTS AND METHODS

1 Quality Assurance and Improvement

Introduction

The Oxford English Dictionary defines quality as a "degree of excellence" or "attribute". Chambers describes it as "that which makes a thing what it is" and Collins "a distinguishing characteristic or attribute, the basic character or nature of something". Commenting on quality specifically in industry, Philip B Crosby observes, "The first erroneous assumption is that quality means goodness, or luxury, or shininess, or weight... If a Cadillac conforms to all the requirements of a Cadillac, then it is a quality car. If a Pinto conforms to all the requirements of a Pinto, then it is a quality car." (Crosby, 1980) Other definitions originating in industry are "fitness for purpose" and "meeting the customer's requirement".

Quality can therefore relate to products, to people or characteristics. These are definitions in neutral terms, but in general, a value judgement is attributed to the concept of quality. When it is said that something or someone has "quality", this is always meant positively.

Learning Outcomes

After studying this chapter the reader should be able to:
− give a definition of quality in general terms;
− understand how standards and criteria can be applied in the commercial world;
− explain the difference between quality assurance and quality improvement;
− give at least two definitions of quality as it is applied to health care;
− describe the areas of care relating to Donabedian's structure, process and outcome standards and criteria;
− discuss the advantages and disadvantages of the methods of assessment mentioned in this chapter;
− describe the two main methods of implementing quality assurance.

The Concept of Quality

The concept of "quality" can often be a subjective one. For instance, when a number of consumers are asked to name the most important characteristics of the car they would like to own, their answers typically refer to reliability, safety, cost, fuel economy, environmental factors, speed, performance, appearance or comfort, and the actual choice of vehicle may range from a Mini to a Rolls-Royce.

In considering the quality of apples, replies may include red or green apples, sweet or sour, firm, crisp or soft, unblemished skin, smell and price; country of origin and place of purchase may also be taken into consideration.

In other words, different characteristics are valued by different people. In both of the examples above, various features or criteria are identified as being the most important ones. The views of quality depend on the values and experiences of the consumer. One individual may choose a car solely on the grounds that it looks good and is fast, while another may consider reliability, fuel economy and environmental factors exclusively. When choosing apples, one person wants red and sweet, another prefers green and sour. How, therefore, can the quality of the car or apple be identified? The answer in regard to the car is to describe standards for both appearance and speed, and also for reliability, fuel economy and environmental factors; or in terms of the apple for red and green, sweet and sour. In short, each criterion can be identified separately, without passing judgement as to whether one condition is better or worse than another.

> **Study Activity 1.**
> Consider a recent experience of your own as a customer of a service. How would you merit it on a scale of 1 to 6? Write down how you are making your judgement. Discuss your experience and what you have written with other members of the group.

The quality of products distinguishes items from each other so that they can be "identified" as jam, champagne, wholemeal bread, unleaded petrol and so on and, as such, they are judged on the basis of their suitability for their intended purpose. In the case of people, the quality is often the result of their education, training and expertise.

In their search for excellence, Peters and Waterman (1982) identified eight attributes which characterised excellent and innovative companies, where chaotic but creative work styles were encouraged in return for quick action and regular experimentation.

The eight attributes are as follows:
– a bias for action; a "do it", "fix it", "try it" philosophy
– close to the customer; constant learning from those they serve
– autonomy and entrepreneurship; encouragement of risk-taking and innovation
– productivity through people; respect for the individual
– hands-on, value-driven; management by walking about (MBWA) looking for evidence of the values of the organisation

- stick to the knitting; staying close to the business known
- simple form, lean staff; structures which are "elegantly simple" with a lean top level
- simultaneous loose–tight properties; autonomy on the shop floor; fanatical about core values; both centralised and decentralised activities are highly valued.

The one condition found over and over again, whether in industry, the commercial world or health care, is that such values, although frequently and simply stated, are rarely lived by.

Many of the concepts underpinning quality and the total quality management approach originate from the foundation literature and work of three of the leading authorities on quality in the USA, W Edwards Deming, P Crosby and J M Juran. The fourteen points in Deming's management agenda (1986) clearly place the responsibility for quality within the sphere of management and give a high value to people and ongoing training. Juran (1988) emphasises the importance of the customer and the need for improving quality by a project-based approach, embracing quality planning, quality control and quality improvement. Crosby's method (1989) is widely used in the UK and his fourteen steps to quality provide a systematic approach to total quality management. The emphasis here is on early commitment at the "top" and total involvement through teamwork.

Standards and Criteria

The conditions which describe quality are known as standards and criteria.

Standards

Collins dictionary defines standard as "a level of excellence or quality" and "an accepted or approved example of something against which others are judged or measured". Both of these definitions tell us something about the meaning of standards in the context of quality assurance: a standard is the level of performance which is generally recognised as being acceptable, adequate, or satisfactory and is used as a benchmark or reference point against which comparisons can be made.

Criteria

If we are going to make a judgement as to whether a standard has or has not been achieved we need something to base the judgement on, items or factors which we can measure. The things which we can measure are known as criteria. They are the separate measurable items which, taken together and scored, form the basis for deciding whether or not the standard has been met.

In order to measure or make an assessment of quality, we need to identify the criteria (i.e. the items we are going to measure) and to agree the standards which we are aiming to achieve (i.e. the accepted, approved level).

It may be helpful to take an example from the commercial world. A product is to

be made and sold, e.g. a tin of beans. The agreed standard which we are aiming to achieve is the production of a successful item with sales of ten million tins per annum. The criteria which will decide whether or not this standard has been achieved are as follows:
- a product which complies with government and EC food regulations
- beans that are acceptable to the customer and have nutritional value
- a reliable and prespecified supply of beans
- an agreed cost of the beans and other ingredients
- an efficient method of processing and canning the beans
- a competitive selling price
- nationwide availability in shops and supermarkets
- efficient marketing and distribution
- ten million tins are bought per annum.

These criteria can be measured, for example, on a scale of one to ten, and whether or not the standard is achieved will depend on how well the criteria score. In Chapter Four the principles of criteria and standard setting will be applied specifically in a nursing context.

> **Study Activity 2.**
> Imagine that you are a travel agent. You want to be able to offer attractive, good-value family holidays in some European country. Construct a standard and a set of criteria to accomplish this and decide which country you are going to choose. Write this all down and discuss in your group.

Quality Assessment

Standards and criteria are used to give an indication of desired quality against which the criteria can be used to gauge actual quality. The measurement takes place by comparing what is desirable against what is actually taking place. This measurement is generally called *quality assessment*. The term *evaluation* is also sometimes used. However, evaluation is generally a more comprehensive study concerned with determining the extent to which a planned intervention achieves predetermined objectives in a systematic and scientific manner.

Quality Assurance and Quality Improvement

The results of the assessment can be used in two ways. Firstly, things which can be regarded as satisfactory may be accepted and maintained. This presupposes that it was "quality" which was defined in the first place. This is called *quality assurance*. For things which turn out to be "unsatisfactory", an attempt at improvement should be made. This is *quality improvement*. Quality assessment should never be carried out as an end in itself. It cannot be isolated from quality assurance and quality improvement. In addition, the assessment and subsequent corrective action need to be undertaken at regular intervals to ensure that systematic quality assurance is being carried out and maintained. As quality systems have developed within health care, the complex, dynamic nature of quality and its measurement, coupled with the inability to *guarantee* a degree of excellence, have led us to talk much more about quality improvement systems and less about quality assurance systems. Some would go so far as to say that assurance is impossible and improvement is a more realistic and accurate description of what actually takes place within health care.

> **Study Activity 3.**
> You are keen to buy an item for recreation, e.g. a badminton racket, hill-walking boots. Write down the criteria you would use to make your purchase, and discuss these in your group.

Quality in Health Care
Beginnings
In health care the concept of quality has always been paramount. How then should it be defined and interpreted? For an explanation of quality specifically related to health care the definitions provided by dictionaries alone are not enough for our purpose.

The earliest written health service records are probably those dating from the Babylonian Empire circa 1700 BC where sanctions are described for providing poor-quality health care. In the Law of Hammurabi, one of the kings of Babylonia, punishments are described which were applied to a doctor who had caused a patient harm.

These punishments were quite uncompromising. For example, article 218 of this law states: "When a doctor has operated on someone using a bronze knife and has thereby caused this person's death, or when he has opened a person's cataract with his bronze knife and has thus ruined the eye, his hand shall be cut off."

The Egyptians in the time of the Pharaohs had a similar system of sanctions for the occasions when a doctor provided poor service. On the other hand, a doctor who gave high-quality care was worshipped like a god. The architect and physician Imhotep, who lived during the Third Dynasty (2750-2680 BC), was such a person. It is notable, however, that nursing is not mentioned anywhere in these ancient sources.

Florence Nightingale, during the course of her duties, gathered together a body of knowledge from which sound judgements could be made. Acting on the findings of her research she introduced standards of infection control which reduced the mortality rate of soldiers during the Crimean War from 42% to 2%. In her *Notes on Nursing: What it is and What it is not*, first published in 1859, she specified explicit standards of nursing care and identified the following as aspects of care which nurses should be monitoring in a systematic way:
– noise and its control around the sick
– consistency in the quality and serving of food

– types of beds, mattresses and bed linen
– the positioning of beds
– airiness and cleanliness of rooms.

The importance of identifying standards in such a manner seems to have been lost for a considerable length of time thereafter, and nursing was not to develop its evaluation skills until nearly a century after such principles were first articulated.

Some Definitions

One of the first definitions of quality specifically in the context of health care was made in 1933 in the United States by Lee and Jones. They equated quality with the application of the skills of modern medical science for the benefit of society as a whole. Quality of care was defined as: "the application of all necessary services of modern scientific medicine to the needs of all people" (Lee and Jones, 1933). Without discussing the significance of this definition in detail, we can see that it is a rather broad one.

A more precise definition of quality was given by the American health insurers, Blue Cross and Blue Shield of Chicago. In 1954 they proposed that quality in relation to the provision of health care should possess five characteristics: it should be *available, acceptable, comprehensive, continuous* and *documented*. Avedis Donabedian has been responsible in the United States for conceiving much of the theoretical basis of quality assurance in health care. He associated the concept of quality with a process of evaluation, defining the quality of care as the conformity between actual care and preset criteria (Donabedian, 1970).

In 1966 he identified three approaches to assessing quality of care relating to the *structure*, the *process* and the *outcome*. Thus, it can be checked whether the working systems and organisation lead to a qualitatively desirable result. This is called structure assessment or evaluation, and structure standards and criteria are needed for this. In addition, a process assessment or process evaluation may be carried out focusing on performance and procedures. Therefore process standards and criteria will have to be developed. Finally, assessment or evaluation might be outcome-oriented. This requires the use of outcome standards and criteria to indicate the result that should eventually be achieved.

There is still much debate over many of the terms used in evaluating quality, and the term "standard" is no exception. Standards have been defined as *summary statements* and alternatively as *precise measures*.

Summary Statements

As broad, descriptive statements they reflect the consensus of a group and "within this definition, 'criteria' become the specific elements of behaviour, performance or clinical status that make up their achievement of the standard." (Kitson and Giebing, 1990). The following organisations have adopted this definition:
– RCN Standards of Care Project
– CBO Nursing Quality Assurance Project
– Joint Commission on the Accreditation of Health Care Organizations (JCAHO)

– American Nurses' Association (ANA)

Figure 1.1.1 shows standards as summary statements.

Standards as Summary Statements

Standard: "a professionally agreed level of (nursing) performance appropriate to the population addressed which is achievable, observable, desirable and measurable".

e.g. Each child undergoing routine surgery will be allocated a qualified nurse responsible for his preoperative care and reduction of unnecessary anxiety associated with the surgical procedure.

Criteria: Measurable elements of the standard.

Structure	Process	Outcome
not less than 1 nurse per 6 occupied beds	primary nurse prepares the child and parents for surgery 12 hours prior to operation	the child experiences minimum distress following surgery

---

Figure 1.1.1 *Standards as Summary Statements*

Precise Measures

An alternative is to define standards as precise measures. The standard, often numerical, is the specific, quantitative measure whilst the criteria are simply items or attributes of quality (Figure 1.1.2). This definition has been adopted by Donabedian (1970), Bloch (1977) and Crow (1981). Further discussion on this topic can be found in Chapter Four.

Standards as Precise Measures

Criteria: attribute of structure, process, outcome

Structure	Process	Outcome
staffing of intensive care	blood transfusion during surgery	case fatality

Standards: specific quantitative measure which defines "goodness"

Structure	Process	Outcome
not less than 1 nurse per 2 occupied beds	not less than 5% and not more than 20% of "average" cases	should not exceed 5% for a specified procedure

Source: Donabedian 1989

Figure 1.1.2 *Standards as Precise Measures*

Dimensions of Quality

Donabedian (1966) proposed that quality of care has three components: the *technical, interpersonal* and *organisational* aspects of care (Figure 1.1.3).

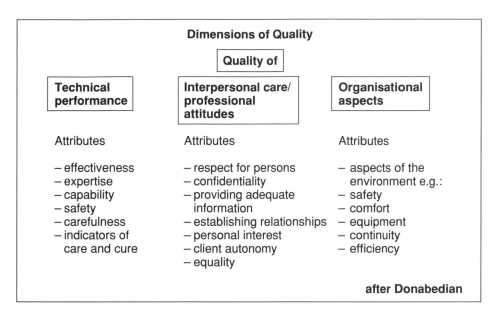

Figure 1.1.3 *Dimensions of Quality*

The quality of *technical* care relates to the ability to achieve the best possible outcome in health care. The *interpersonal* aspect of health care is concerned with the privileged relationship between patient and practitioner, and the trusting, private context within which this takes place. The *organisational* aspects of the quality of care refer to the *amenities*, i.e. the comforts, the convenience to the patient of time and place, the resources and the setting where care takes place.

Maxwell (1984) defines quality care as having six elements or dimensions which require to be held in balance.

effectiveness	– the service achieves the intended benefit for the individual and for the population
efficiency	– resources are not wasted on one service or patient to the detriment of another
equity	– there is a fair share for all the population
accessibility	– services are not compromised by undue limits of time or distance
acceptability	– services are provided such as to satisfy the reasonable expectations of patients, providers and the community
relevance to need	– the service or procedure is what the population or individual actually needs

Study Activity 4.

Consider the closure of a small community hospital and the centralising of services into a district general hospital. In the light of Maxwell's dimensions of quality
a. which dimensions are being increased?
b. which dimensions are being decreased?

Quality Assurance in Health Care

Many activities assess or regulate the quality of care but unless they include efforts to improve quality when necessary they are not quality assurance activities. At its simplest, quality assurance is about describing, measuring and taking action, three distinct phases (Figure 1.1.4).

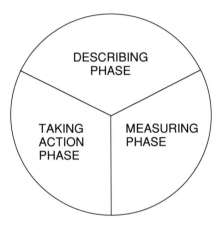

Figure 1.1.4 *The Quality Assurance Cycle*

Quality assurance carries with it a commitment to respond positively to results obtained from an evaluation or assessment. These two key concepts (assessment and commitment to improve if necessary) are illustrated in Williamson's (1982) definition where quality assurance is seen as: "the measurement of the actual level of the service provided plus the efforts to modify when necessary the provision of these services in the light of the results of the measurement". Schroeder (1991) states that: "...as health-care professionals have gained experience in the process of monitoring and evaluation, several consistent premises can be identified as differentiating successful from unsuccessful approaches. Success in this instance is determined by the yielding of useful results that lead to improvements in care and practice."

When standards for nursing practice are specified, only then can *actual* nursing practice be measured against these. Those aspects of nursing practice which do not meet the preset criteria need to be improved. A structured and systematic method of quality improvement can only be achieved when assessment is carried out at regular intervals and is an integral part of professional practice.

Definitions of Quality Care

Quality of care is:

a. the application of all necessary services of modern scientific medicine to the needs of all people   (1933 Lee & Jones)
b. the degree to which care is available, acceptable, comprehensive, continuous and documented   (1958 Blue Cross)
c. the conformity between actual care and preset criteria   (1970 Donabedian)
d. effective health care to improve the health status and satisfaction of a population within the resources society and individuals have chosen to spend for that care   (1974 Williamson)
e. multidimensional and complex   (1976 Brook)

After Reerink (CBO), The Netherlands

Figure 1.1.5 *Definitions of Quality Care*

Figure 1.1.5 lists some of the definitions that have been given for quality assurance since the first 1933 definition made by Lee and Jones. Such definitions are useful in helping us to formulate ways of thinking about quality of care. However, in order to define precise elements of care, we need to pursue many issues further, and the next section will look at some of the terminology which is most commonly used when referring to the organisation and implementation of quality assurance activity in relation to health care.

Since quality assurance and quality improvement are concerned with describing, measuring and taking action, it may be useful at this point to pause and consider two frequently used terms which the reader may find confusing. These are the terms *monitoring* and *audit.*

Monitoring
Schroeder (1991) has defined monitoring as: "The systematic and ongoing collection and organisation of data related to the indicators of the quality and appropriateness of important aspects of care and the comparison of cumulative data with thresholds for evaluation related to each indicator".

Audit
One generally accepted definition of audit is: "The systematic, critical analysis of the quality of clinical care. This includes the procedures used for diagnosis and treatment, the associated use of resources, and the effect of care on the outcome and quality of life for the patient." (The Health Service, 1989). Norman and Redfern (1993) describe audit in a recent paper as "the measurement necessary to provide practitioners with information on whether improvement is required". The term audit is at times used simply for the collection of information, the measurement phase of the quality assurance cycle. At other times its definition embraces a commitment to change or improvement.

The context and strategic direction within which such activity takes place must also be considered and it may be worth while taking time to look briefly at two other frequently used terms, *Total Quality Management (TQM)* and *Continuous Quality Improvement (CQI)*.

TQM is based on an enabling philosophy which is totally committed to quality and which emphasises teamwork and participation of all employees. It requires commitment to the marketplace and customer, and is management-led. TQM demands a change in the culture of the organisation and by doing so it seeks to release the organisational potential for continuous quality improvement (CQI) which emphasises the dynamic and ongoing nature of achieving quality.

What should not be forgotten is that quality embraces the individual's total experience of the health services provided. This includes the physical environment and the amenities provided, the appropriateness of support arrangements and the effectiveness of delivery of the care and treatment, to the final outcome in terms of health gain. Monitoring and audit will be considered in more detail in Chapters Three and Four.

The Organisation of Quality Assurance

Quality assurance can be organised in a variety of ways:
– according to the people who are taking part
– by the way the assessment is undertaken
– by the method that is used for the implementation of quality assurance.

When quality assurance is carried out by staff of one service only, nursing for example, then it is defined as *uniprofessional*. When it is carried out by staff from various services working together, for example medical, nursing and paramedical staff, then it is known as *interprofessional* implementation.

It is important to bear in mind that quality improvement in nursing practice is only part of an overall strategy and programme towards quality improvement in health care. A patient-centred approach must always put the patient first. This requires interprofessional activity, as professionals in this situation should not be working in isolation.

On the other hand, there has to be room for putting one's own house in order and therefore the composition of the group should be dictated by the complexity of the issue being addressed. For instance, a quality improvement activity to improve pain management, if patient-centred, should include in the group other key players such as a doctor, a physiotherapist and patient representation.

Methods of Assessment

There are several options regarding the assessment of quality assurance activity. These are dependent on when the assessment is undertaken and who carries out the assessment.

Retrospective Assessment

The quality of nursing care can be assessed after the cycle of care has been completed, for instance through the examination of nursing records. This assessment reviews the delivery of nursing care after it has taken place and as it has been documented in the records. This method of assessment is therefore retrospective, i.e. "after the event", as for example in Phaneuf's Audit. Traditionally, a retrospective examination of records has played a large part in the definition of the term "audit". This would be in line with the popular conception of audit, as in a financial audit of company accounts.

Concurrent Assessment

Nursing performance can also be assessed while care is taking place. It is therefore being examined concurrently, i.e. "at the time of the event".

Prospective Assessment

Finally, the quality of nursing care can be assessed in advance of the caring process. Before nursing intervention, a statement is made as to the anticipated, desirable outcome in terms of standards and criteria. It is therefore prospective, i.e. "before the event". The actual outcome of the performance cannot be measured properly until later.

The advantages and disadvantages of these three methods are shown in Figure 1.1.6.

RETROSPECTIVE	CONCURRENT	PROSPECTIVE
quick	time-consuming	quick
potential for inaccurate record of actual care	actual care observed	potential for inaccuracies
inexpensive	expensive	inexpensive
discrepancies identified cannot be rectified	discrepancies identified can be rectified while the patient is still in care	discrepancies identified can be rectified before care is delivered

Figure1.1.6 *Advantages and Disadvantages of Retrospective, Concurrent and Prospective Assessment*

Internal Assessment

Internal quality assurance means that the assessment is made in-house with staff themselves determining the quality standards. They also implement the methods to establish and improve these standards. Emphasis is increasingly being placed on peer review as a valuable form of assessment, where quality of nursing performance is appraised by fellow practising nurses.

External Assessment

External methods which assist in the regulation of standards within the United Kingdom include visits from and recommendations by the Hospital Advisory Service and the Mental Welfare Commission. Inspection visits by the National Boards to colleges of health studies help to maintain the required educational standards. The implementation of Project 2000 has meant that new regulatory methods of both internal and external assessment and evaluation have been introduced, with the responsibility being placed at local level. More recently the King's Fund Accreditation Programme for Organisational Audit has been implemented to monitor standards in hospitals.

Methods of Implementation

Centrally Organised Implementation

Central implementation means that quality assurance is carried out from one point within the whole organisation by specially appointed staff or by a committee which has been specifically set up to implement quality assurance. This might be an identified quality assurance department. Apart from being responsible for quality assurance in nursing, such a department might also engage in quality assurance within other disciplines or the organisation as a whole.

The main features of the centrally organised method are:
- nursing care is assessed from an overview,"a skim over the surface"
- the method of assessment is prescribed
- the instrument for measuring quality is predetermined
- the staff who are carrying out nursing care are not normally involved with the implementation of quality assurance and do not bear responsibility for it.

Locally Organised Implementation

In the case of locally organised methods, quality assurance can be carried out within each section of the organisation. Working committees comprise the staff from within a department or unit. These committees implement quality assurance in close collaboration with the other staff of the department or unit. All of the employees are responsible for the implementation and the progress of the quality assurance programme in their area.

The main features of the locally organised method are:
- the assessment is small-scale and subject-based
- the instrument used for measuring quality is determined within the department or unit
- the staff responsible for the nursing care are closely involved in the implementation of quality assurance.

> **Study Activity 5.**
> Discuss in your group which other participants apart from the nurse(s) are needed to ensure the successful implementation of a quality assurance programme in health care.

Conclusion

Even in the relatively short time that quality assurance methods and systems have been implemented in the delivery of health care, changes in terminology and approaches have abounded. For example, the current fashion is to favour the term "quality improvement" rather than "quality assurance". In a similar vein, many of those involved in quality strategy now prefer to use the term "continuous quality improvement" (CQI) rather than "total quality management" (TQM). In view of all this, the reader should not be too concerned if the terminology used in this book is not consistent with their own previous understanding of quality assurance terminology.

Perhaps this chapter should have been subtitled "Clarity and Confusion". It has been many people's experience that just when you think you've got it, you lose it! Any definitions of quality, quality assurance, quality improvement, audit, standard setting and monitoring have a kaleidoscopic nature - colourful, cloudy, clear, and ever-changing. Many attempts have been made to define such concepts. Norman and Redfern (1993) put it very well:

"What is immediately striking on entering the quality arena is the lack of consistency in the way in which common terms are used in the voluminous literature. Ninety-six terms for the review of care can be derived by combining either 'medical', 'health', 'clinical' or 'professional' with 'care', 'activity', 'standards', or 'quality' and with either 'assessment', 'evaluation', 'assurance', 'audit', 'monitoring' or 'review'. ...This confusion in terminology may be partly the result of the rapid expansion of interest in quality and quality assurance in health care, as a result of which a number of terms have become current before their meaning is clear."

But how interchangeable are such words as "monitor", "assess", "audit" and "evaluate"? When confused, go to the dictionary.
Clarify your own understanding.
Share your meaning in discussion.
Seek clarification from others.
"Hang on" and dont get "hung up".

This chapter has looked at a number of definitions and has, we hope, helped to demystify some of the jargon likely to be encountered in the process of becoming familiar with quality in health care.

References

Bloch D 1977 *Criteria, standards, norms - crucial terms in quality assurance.* Journal of Nursing Administration, 7(7): September: 20 30.
Crow R 1981 *Research and standards of nursing care.* Journal of Advanced Nursing, 6: 491-496.
Crosby P B 1980 Quality is Free: The Art of Making Quality Certain. Mentor, New York.
Crosby P B 1989 Let's Talk Quality. McGraw-Hill, New York.
Deming W E 1986 Out of the Crisis. MIT Center for Advanced Engineering Studies, Boston.
Department of Health 1990 Working for Patients. HMSO, London.

Department of Health 1991 Caring for People. HMSO, London.

Donabedian A 1966 *Evaluating the quality of medical care.* Millbank Memorial Fund Quarterly, 44: 166-203.

Donabedian A 1970 *Patient care evaluation.* Hospitals, April: 131-136.

Griffiths E R 1984 NHS Management Report. HMSO, London.

Juran J M 1988 Juran on Planning for Quality. Free Press, New York.

Kitson A L and Giebing H 1990 Nursing Quality Assurance in Practice. RCN/CBO, London, Utrecht (unpublished).

Lee R I and Jones L W 1933 The Fundamentals of Good Medical Care. University of Chicago Press, Chicago.

Maxwell R J 1984 *Quality assessment in health.* British Medical Journal, 288: 1470-1472.

Nightingale F 1859 Notes on Nursing: What it is and What it is not. Harrison & Sons, London.

Norman I J and Redfern S J 1993 *The quality of nursing.* Nursing Times, Vol. 89, No 27: 7 July: 40-43.

Peters T J and Waterman Jr R H 1982 In Search of Excellence. Harper and Row, New York.

Schroeder P 1991 The Encyclopedia of Nursing Care Quality. Aspen Publishers, Gaithersburg, MD.

Medical Audit, Scottish Working Paper 2 1989 Working for Patients. The Health Service, Edinburgh.

Williamson J W 1982 Teaching Quality Assurance–Cost Containment in Health Care. Jossey Bass, London.

World Health Organization 1985 Targets for Health For All. WHO Regional Office for Europe, Copenhagen.

Further Reading

Frederick B J, Sharp J O and Atkins N 1988 *Quality of patient care: whose decision....Consumer or health care professional?* Journal of Nursing Quality Assurance, May, 2 (3): 1-10.

Koch H 1991 Total Quality Management in Health Care. Longman, Harlow.

Oakland J S 1989 Total Quality Management. Heinemann, Oxford.

Reid E 1988 *An overview of quality assurance: the concept and the reality.* Recent Advances in Nursing (19): 64-67.

Shaw C D 1986 Introducing Quality Assurance. King's Fund, Paper No. 64, London.

Scottish Enterprise 1991 A Guide to Total Quality Management. Scottish Enterprise, Glasgow.

Walton M 1989 The Deming Management Method. Mercury Books, London.

Wilson C R M 1987 Hospital-Wide Quality Assurance. Models for Implementation and Development. W B Saunders, Philadelphia.

2 Professional Practice

Introduction

This chapter addresses a number of key issues which contribute to the planning and delivery of excellence in nursing and the context within which care takes place. As individuals, we reach conclusions based on personal experience and expectations; in addition we may identify common principles and values to reflect a community's shared beliefs about the essential worth of health care. At the same time, as medical, paramedical or nursing professionals, we make judgements based on our profession's values and beliefs, its code of ethics and the professional standards it has established. In making judgements we can consider episodes or events in isolation or we may compare two or more events or situations in order to draw conclusions. In a more general sense, the quality of health care reflects the values of society, professional groups and individual practitioners and relies on a shared understanding and acceptance of those important principles that reflect a quality service.

Learning Outcomes

After studying this chapter the reader should be able to:
- explain how a nursing model can contribute to good practice;
- list current official publications which provide the guiding principles for nursing's beliefs and practices;
- describe the role and function of the nurse;
- explain the aims of *The Patient's Charter*;
- describe the named nurse concept;
- describe the measures which need to be taken in order to implement the named nurse concept;
- describe the systems for organising care.

Quality of Nursing Care

Schroeder (1991) suggests that: "Today's view of quality then, incorporates knowledge, skills and behaviors of practitioners, as well as use of patient, physician and payer measures of quality." When defining quality nursing care it is important to take account of the underlying values and beliefs of nurses and the way they organise nursing care. In essence, quality of care in a technically orientated, task allocation setting may be defined quite differently from quality care within an area delivering primary nursing. In a needs-based but task-orientated system,

25

there will rarely be time for a more holistic type of nursing and there is the probability that nursing methods may well reflect procedures and techniques rather than interpersonal and contextual issues related to quality of care.

The choice of either a needs-based or an interactionist approach will depend to a large extent on the model of nursing that is being followed. Nursing models are attempts to make an explicit framework for the concept of nursing and to describe the relationships between the nurse, humanity, the environment and health. "In nursing practice, models can be used to develop assessment tools, care plans and outcome criteria. They provide frameworks for the philosophy and objectives of a nursing department. The nursing process, standards of practice and quality assurance issues are promoted." (Herbert, 1988) There are a variety of nursing models being used, each with its own mission for nursing, each requiring its own assessment tool. (Figure 1.2.1)

Conceptual Framework for Nursing (after Meleis 1985) **Characteristics of Main Approaches**		
Needs-based	**Interactionist**	**Outcome**
problem-focused	nursing as interpersonal process	focus on identifying outcome of nursing care
focus on nurse's functions	nurse must clarify own values	recognises interdependence of nurse and client
reductionist approach	nurse uses self in therapeutic way	client assessed within context
illness-based	care is humanistic not mechanistic	recognises harmony with environment homeostasis
illness defined as deviation to be corrected	illness defined as inevitable from which experience can grow	incorporates needs-based and interactionist approaches

Figure1.2.1 Conceptual Framework for Nursing

One of the criticisms made about nursing models is that they are too complex and too theoretical. However, "If all this talk of nursing models leads nurses to clarify their own beliefs about their work, increases their ability to discuss issues involving personal and political attitudes with more openness, and helps them become more professionally accountable for their actions, then we are getting somewhere." (Salvage, 1985)

Accountability

Nurses, midwives and health visitors are required to be "personally accountable" for their practice and, in the exercise of their professional accountability, must act in accordance with the sixteen clauses which provide the standards and framework for the nursing profession as stated in the *Code of Professional Conduct* (1992). Experience has shown that involvement in quality assurance programmes has "...benefits beyond the identification of errors. Nurses can be empowered to be accountable for the practice of excellent nursing care using quality assurance monitoring as a tool for identifying opportunities to improve patient care." (Schroeder, 1991)

The implementation of quality assurance programmes can contribute significantly to professional development. Schroeder (1991) states that: "Nurses involved in quality assurance are required to:
– conduct insightful assessments of their areas of practice while researching and writing a scope of care
– demonstrate accountability as they determine aspects of patient care that are essential to their areas of expertise
– apply basic research techniques as data-gathering strategies are designed and conducted
– communicate with peers and colleagues in other disciplines as the results of quality assurance activities are analyzed and reported throughout the organization."

Accountability in nursing practice must be able to depend on accountability in management, thus the Audit Commission underlines the importance of maintaining and improving standards in a report on making the best use of ward resources: "Nursing is too important a component of patient care and of hospital budgets to be left to develop in isolation. The commitment of general managers and doctors in management, as well as managers of nursing services, to an agreed vision and strategy for the development of nursing services is vital." (1991)

In order to accomplish this "vision" the participation of all staff is essential. In support of this view, Schroeder (1991) cites at least six authors who have highlighted the value of "involving the bedside practitioners in the conduct of quality assurance". The very nature of the environment of practising nurses creates flexibility and innovation which can only benefit the challenge of the quality assurance programme and provide opportunities for improvements in quality of care. Unfortunately, however, the resources are not always there to see this through in practice and nurses are finding themselves increasingly stretched to meet the growing demands of patients and purchasers.

It is now a well-established fact that nursing is by far the largest Item in a hospital's budget. This one item alone accounts for over one-third of health boards'/authorities' revenue expenditure, and consumes 3% of all public expenditure. In addition to this, nurses exercise control over a considerable amount of hospital expenditure. In the light of this, it is imperative that there is effective and efficient use of such resources.

> **Study Activity 1.**
> Discuss ways in which participating in quality assurance activity can increase your personal and professional accountability.

The Role and Function of the Nurse

Historically, it has been extremely difficult to define the role and function of the professional nurse, with a certain amount of confusion and a lack of clarity surrounding the role. Furthermore, "good" nursing has often been described as invisible and only obvious by its absence. Much has been written about the invisibility of nursing and the critical differences identified in skilled nursing care as a consequence of the cognitive and interpretative skills of the expert nurse. "So much of what nurses do is invisible. Good nursing care is often demonstrated by the fact that you can't see it. In units caring for elderly people, where good nursing is being provided, the place looks ordinary. People are well dressed and comfortable, undertaking as much as possible for themselves, and living in a setting which is full of home comforts. This cannot be achieved without skill and experience in nursing elderly people. Privacy and dignity of patients or residents are maintained by making it look as if they are not being nursed." (RCN, 1992)

Describing this intangible nature of nursing, Benner (1984) states how the knowledge embedded in actual nursing practice has gone "uncharted and unstudied". The failure to systematically and cumulatively examine such practice closely "has deprived nursing theory of the uniqueness and richness of the knowledge embedded in expert clinical practice".

Changes in health care delivery such as community care, *The Patient's Charter* (1991), the increased number of day surgeries, and changes in clinical practice mean that the role of the nurse is constantly under review. To patients receiving skilled care, the value of nursing is self-evident. However, with the ever-increasing pressure on budgets to provide a cost-effective service, the benefits of expenditure on nursing care are being questioned. The NHS reforms, with the separation of purchaser and provider, have led to a greater awareness of costs which may result in, for example, an effort to cut back on full-time, permanent nursing staff despite the fact that there is a growing body of research which shows a direct link between the employment of qualified nurses and the quality of patient care.

> **Study Activity 2.**
>
> Explain why it is difficult to quantify the various elements of good nursing practice.

A recent study undertaken by the University of York (Carr-Hill et al, 1992) set out to "examine the links between inputs into the process of nursing, in particular, the skill mix of nursing staff and the outputs of nursing in terms of the quality and outcome of care". The results of the research are that "In general ...grade mix had an effect on the quality of care in so far as the quality of care was better the higher the grade (and skill) of the nurses who provided it, but the variation in the quality of care between the different grades of staff was reduced when higher graded staff worked in combination with lower graded staff."

The Role and Function of the Professional Nurse (1992) sets out to identify and clarify those aspects which distinguish professional nursing practice from care given by people who do not have a professional nursing qualification. It will only be with an understanding of this that the most efficient and effective employment and deployment of nursing staff will be possible.

These roles and functions are described under six headings:
- the planning of nursing required for each individual patient
- the delivery of direct care
- identifying when it is appropriate for the nursing care of patients to be undertaken by those without a professional nursing qualification
- preparing and supporting those who do not have a professional nursing qualification to undertake such activities as are delegated to them by the professional nurse
- the effective and efficient management and organisation of resources of personnel, equipment and services directly controlled or requisitioned by the professional nurse
- standard setting, nursing audit and clinical audit.

> **Study Activity 3.**
> Write down in your own words the three most important responsibilities that qualified nurses have which should not be undertaken by unqualified staff. Discuss your choices in your group.

Strategy for Nursing, Midwifery and Health Visiting

One very important document which must not be allowed to gather dust on a shelf is the *Strategy for Nursing, Midwifery and Health Visiting (Scotland)* (1990). Commitment and consultation were encouraged from the start of its development among nurses throughout the country. Subsequently, action plans were developed at organisational and clinical levels to ensure progress in its implementation.

The document was sent out to every practising nurse, midwife and health visitor by the Department of Health, Nursing Division, and its aim was to address the changes which face the profession over the next decade. The strategy document outlines four main areas where change is considered necessary in the form of key objectives:
- nursing practice
- nurse management
- education for nursing
- nursing research.

The strategy helps us, as a profession and as individuals, to take a fresh look at all of these areas, reappraising outmoded objectives, policies and procedures. Instead of the attitude "We have always done it like that", it encourages the attitude "How can we do it better?" or "Can we achieve an improved outcome by changing the way we work?" In short, by meeting the challenges and targets identified in the document, nurses will not only improve the quality of care that they provide, but will also raise their professional standing through education, training and research.

The Nursing Standard of Care

Respect for the whole person. It is necessary to be aware of each person's capacity, concerns and expectations, as well as their health problems; and to acknowledge their spiritual needs and aspirations, and their right to live to their full potential.
Respect for the individual. All staff should be sensitive to the wide variation in individual characters, circumstances, values and cultural background.
Respect for dignity and self-esteem. People have a right to expect honesty, respect and the preservation of their dignity.

The Patient's Charter 1991

Figure 1.2.2 *The Nursing Standard of Care*

Universal Standard

The strategy outlines an expression of values which are the foundation of nursing, midwifery and health visiting practice. These values relate both to patients as recipients of nursing and to nurses as providers of care. Three of the eight values (Figure 1.2.2) expressed within this philosophy of nursing are fundamental patient-related values and these were subsequently adopted as a universal standard within *The Patient's Charter* (1991). The Charter states that: "A universal standard of care has been developed by nurses. It expresses the way that everyone at every stage can reasonably expect to be treated. From today, it is being adopted throughout the NHS."

The Patient's Charter

The Department of Health's *The Patient's Charter, A Charter for Health* (1991), which outlines the Government's commitment to the rights of the public and the consumer, took effect in April 1992 and has preceded and pre-empted similar but more localised standards and targets within health care departments.

The Patient's Charter is part of *The Citizen's Charter* and is an attempt to explain what the public can expect from the National Health Service and what they are entitled to. It sets out the Government's commitment :
– to improve quality at all levels
– to increase choice to the consumer
– to publish NHS standards of performance
– to make it easier to complain when these standards are not
  achieved
– to improve value for money by improving quality.

At a national level, in order to ensure its implementation, *The Patient's Charter* was accompanied by the *Framework for Action,* a detailed action plan for meeting Charter requirements. These documents were published following wide

consultation with the public and professionals. *Framework for Action* outlines a programme of action for:
– improving health
– improving care for patients
– empowering staff.

Following on from the national Charter, purchasers and providers are publishing their own charters with specific guarantees to users of the health services. Such charters are widely distributed locally; they seek to identify the issues of local importance and are updated regularly.

It is hoped that this sharing of knowledge and standards will empower patients to play an active part in their care, treatment and in the promotion of their health. The Charter has opened doors to the public to "tell us what you think" and has therefore made it easier to identify the quality issues important at least to those who are speaking out at this time. The Charter has also made explicit the purpose and values of the NHS in Scotland (Figure 1.2.3).

The Values of the NHS in Scotland are:

- to provide fair entitlement and access to its services
- to identify and seek to meet people's needs and wishes
- to set out to achieve the highest standards possible
  – of care and respect for each person
  – of results
  – of value for money
- to improve standards through research, education, monitoring and review *while enabling those who work in the Service*
- to achieve its purpose
- to share its values
  and
- to feel valued themselves.

Figure 1.2.3 *The Values of the NHS in Scotland*

The Named Nurse

One of the most innovative and consequential features in the Department of Health's Charter is the concept of a named nurse for each patient. In response to the announcement of the named nurse concept, local health charters have made a commitment to this particular charter standard, namely, that patients should have a named, qualified nurse, midwife or health visitor who is to be responsible for their nursing or midwifery care.

The named nurse initiative firmly places the responsibility for a patient's care with a single person, the named nurse. This approach should provide greater autonomy and accountability for the practising nurse, promote maximum continuity and co-ordination of care for the patient and extend consumer rights.

Patient-centred care should underpin the named nurse concept

- the named nurse will be a qualified nurse
- the ward should already be operating a patient-centred approach to organising patient care
- there should be continuity, with the same nurse being allocated to the same patient on a regular basis
- the named nurse should see each patient for whom she is responsible every time she is on duty and should be available for discussion
- the named nurse should co-ordinate the planning, delivery and evaluation of care for all patients within her care group
- the patient's wishes as to who his named nurse is should be respected
- the named nurse should be identifiable to the patient and his family
- the named nurse should introduce herself to the patient and provide information regarding her responsibilities in respect of his care
- the named nurse should be seen as a quality target and a right of patients
- this standard should be monitored on a regular basis to plot progress or identify stumbling-blocks to its successful implementation.

Making the patient aware of his named nurse

- the patient should receive written notification on admission of who his named nurse is, with an explanation of what this means
- the named nurse should be identified by name on all nursing documentation and care plans
- patients should always know the name of the nurse who will take over in the named nurse's absence
- copies of duty rotas should be placed in the ward area to inform patients when their named nurse is next on duty
- name badges should be worn by all staff members.

In order to act as a named nurse the nurse needs to have:

- the freedom to exercise accountability and autonomy in practice within the boundaries of her professional knowledge
- complete managerial and educational support so that she is empowered to practise in this way
- confidence and interpersonal skills to form the necessary relationship with patients, their carers, and the multiprofessional team
- support in monitoring, maintaining and developing standards of practice
- a working environment with the agreed proportions of qualified and support staff to deliver this approach
- opportunities for continued personal, professional development and support
- a manageable caseload of patients
- the opportunity to give enough direct patient care to form a therapeutic relationship with the patient
- the ability to help other nurses develop their named nurse approach
- the ability to work in partnership with other nurses, acting on their behalf when necessary
- awareness of different ways of organising care.

Adapted from *Issues in Nursing and Health No. 14*, RCN, 1992.

In order to introduce the named nurse it is suggested that in the first instance the ward/department charge nurse could be the named nurse. This is already the case to some extent in current and past practice, particularly where care is not yet organised in a primary nurse or key worker system. This may need to happen where there are few qualified nurses or where staff are, as yet, ill prepared to fulfil the role of named nurse.

However, this is a transitional stage and should not be seen as an end in itself. Successful implementation of this approach needs careful preparation of patients, nurses, and the interprofessional team, and a long-term strategy of support, development and the management of change. It is suggested that each area develops criteria for the standard that *each patient has a named nurse who is responsible for his care.* Figure 1.2.4 gives an example of a standard which can be adapted for local use.

Broadly speaking, implementation of the named nurse concept falls into at least three areas: *courtesy, information* and *organisation of work.*

Courtesy and Information
These two aspects should have already been addressed in the implementation of local charters. The name of the responsible nurse should be made readily available to patients and relatives by means of business cards, information booklets, name badges and photographs of staff on duty. Unfortunately, such trimmings are easy to implement without much understanding of, or commitment to, the principles which underpin the concept of the named nurse, i.e. personal and professional accountability in a patient-centred care setting.

Organisation of Work
Patient care needs to be organised to promote continuity and co-ordination, and therefore promote quality. Some systems of organising care are more conducive to the therapeutic values of nursing but there is no single correct way of organising nursing care delivery for all settings. It is the responsibility of each nursing team to make an informed judgement in the choice of the system which is most appropriate to the needs of their patients and clients.

Study Activity 4.

Using your own experience, describe how the named nurse initiative is being implemented in the clinical area with which you are most familiar.

a. What is the evidence that the initiative has been implemented?

b. Does the evidence suggest that the essence of the initiative has been grasped, or is it only the trimmings?

c. What preparation and training is being given to nurses?

d. How is the implementation being monitored?

Figure 1.2.4 *The Named Nurse Initiative*

Standard Reg. No.	Draft Standard (Suggestion for adaptation)	Achieve Standard By
Topic	Accountability	Review Standard By
Sub-Topic	Named Nurse	Signature of Director of Quality
Care Group	All Patients and Clients	
Source of Production		
Adopted By/Adapted By		
Rationale	To provide greater continuity of care for patients and accountability for nurses.	
Standard Statement	Each patient has a named qualified nurse who is responsible for his care.	

STRUCTURE	PROCESS	OUTCOME
Each nurse has access to information on the named nurse initiative.	A care co-ordinator identifies a named nurse for each patient.	Accountability is formally located for each patient's care with a nurse by name.
Systems are in place to prepare and inform the patients, nurses and interprofessional team of the named nurse concept.	The nurse introduces herself and informs the patient of her role as named nurse.	Each patient/relative can identify a nurse responsible for his care.
There is evidence of: management support; a working environment with the agreed proportions of qualified and support staff; professional knowledge, skills and confidence to act as a named nurse.	The nurse ensures that, when she is absent, care is handed over to an identified person.	The nurse responsible for care is identified within nursing documentation.
	The nurse identifies herself by name on all documentation and care plans.	Continuity of care is maintained.
The named nurse has a manageable caseload which is specified.	The nurse carrying out any aspect of care introduces herself to the patient.	The chosen method of care delivery is identifiable.
Work is organised to facilitate the named nurse approach.	The named nurse manages, co-ordinates and delegates care and takes opportunities to form a therapeutic relationship with the patient.	
Photographs/name badges/information booklets or business cards in use to inform patients/relatives.	The named nurse works in partnership with other nurses acting on their behalf when necessary.	

Systems for Organising Care

Primary nursing

Primary nursing is seen as the most highly developed form of named nursing and is very specific about levels of accountability and organisation. It is a professional model of practice in which a qualified nurse is responsible and accountable for the nursing care of a small caseload of patients for the entire duration of their care. In reality, many clinical areas do not have professionals in sufficient numbers to adopt this approach. In these situations this pure form of nursing is seen as a long-term goal rather than an immediate realistic outcome.

Key Workers

Key workers operate in a similar way to primary nurses but may be drawn from the entire interprofessional team. The team decides which member would be most appropriate to co-ordinate care for an individual client.

Case Management

Case management can be seen as the next step after primary nursing. The basic principles are the same but the environment is less restricted. In the case management system the nurse manages the patient's care as his primary nurse from the patient's first contact with the service, (usually visiting the patient's GP) until the patient is discharged from the service. The case manager may also have responsibility for the management of resources.

Patient Allocation

The nurse is assigned a caseload of patients for the duration of her span of duty. Nurses are responsible for carrying out the nursing care for that caseload, with assistance for the elements of care beyond their capabilities. The aim of this system is to give total care to a group of patients for a designated period of time. Whilst this does attempt to individualise care, continuity is sacrificed as a result of the shift system.

Team Nursing

Team nursing is based on the belief that a small group of nurses working together, led by one nurse, can give better care than if they work individually. It uses the skills of all team members so that, in theory, the patients get the best care available. This small team is responsible and accountable for the group of patients allocated to them for their entire hospital stay. There are three prerequisites for team nursing:
– each team is led by a registered nurse, who must have leadership and management skills
– there must be effective written and verbal communication
the style of management must support the role of the team leader.

One method of organising care, *task allocation*, is unacceptable in the promotion of the named nurse concept. This method entails allocating responsibility for carrying out delegated tasks common to all patients. It is a way of organising staff that ensures at least that the minimum standard of physical care is achieved throughout the ward. Task allocation, however, also ensures that care is fragmented and by its very nature results in the denial of the individual's need for holistic care.

Adapted from *Issues in Nursing and Health No. 13,* RCN, 1992.

Like all new and far-reaching developments, the introduction of the named nurse has extensive implications for managerial and educational support if it is to be developed in a meaningful way and not just on paper or in name only.

> **Study Activity 5.**
> Consider from your own experience the ways you have seen nursing care organised, and relate it to how the organisation of work has been described above.

Quality and Professional Practice

Quality assurance must be oriented towards improving the quality of professional practice by nurses for the benefit of patients. The process of standard setting using a patient-centred, dynamic approach does just that. Smith (in Schroeder, 1991) exhorts nurses to "document and articulate their role in the delivery of health-care services to patients and be prepared to identify readily the impact of nursing care on interventions in achieving desired patient outcomes".

Quality assurance is a concept which embraces all of nursing. It should be applied not just to the actual performance of nurses, but also to the environment where care takes place and the conditions in which it happens. At the same time, quality assurance offers the possibility of self-assessing and peer review for improving individual performance. This can be done, for example, by indicating the standards and criteria which should be met and by stating the means that may be used to achieve these. Thus, quality conditions can be set for targets and performance.

One point to bear in mind, however, is that quality assurance that focuses only on the individual performance of a nurse is falling short of its potential usefulness. Quality assurance is certainly not a method of rooting out bad apples and should not be seen as a means of implementing staff appraisal. On its own this would lead to a system of performance evaluation which would miss its principal target of improving the quality of the whole of professional practice. Quality improvement, appraisal and development should work symbiotically to produce a better nurse, a better patient.

Conclusion

Wherever quality assurance takes place, experience tells us that nurses do not regard it as a threat; rather they see it as a necessary and useful part of their job. This is not only because their own role in nursing can be clarified, but also because quality assurance can clearly indicate what nurses *would like to* take responsibility for and what they *are able to* take responsibility for. It sets the boundaries, as it were, within which nurses can guarantee the quality of their professional practice.

References

Audit Commission 1991 The Virtue of Patients. Department of Health, London.

Benner P 1984 From Novice to Expert. Addison-Wesley, Menlo Park, CA.

Carr-Hill R, Dixon R, Gibbs I 1992 Skill Mix and the Effectiveness of Nursing Care. University of York, York.

Herbert M 1988 *The Value of Nursing Models.* Canadian Nurse, Vol. 84, No. 11: 32-34.

Kitson A L 1989 A Framework for Quality: A Patient Centred Approach to Quality Assurance in Health Care. Scutari, Harrow.

NHS in Scotland 1991 The Patient's Charter, A Charter for Health. The Scottish Office, Edinburgh.

Royal College of Nursing 1992 Issues in Nursing and Health, Nos. 13 and 14. RCN, London.

Royal College of Nursing 1992 The Value of Nursing. RCN, London.

UKCC 1992 Code of Professional Conduct (3rd edition). UKCC, London.

Salvage J 1985 The Politics of Nursing. Heinemann, Oxford.

Schroeder P 1991 The Encyclopedia of Nursing Care Quality. Aspen Publishers, Gaithersburg, MD.

Scottish Home and Health Department 1990 Strategy for Nursing, Midwifery and Health Visiting. HMSO, Edinburgh.

Scottish Office 1991 Framework for Action. Scottish Office, Edinburgh.

Scottish Office 1992 The Role and Function of the Professional Nurse. Scottish Home and Health Department, Edinburgh.

Further Reading

Basford L, Slevin O D'A et al 1994 Theory and Practice of Nursing. Campion Press, Edinburgh.

Dimond B 1994 *Standard setting and litigation.* British Journal of Nursing Vol. 3 No. 5: 235-38.

Hancock C *The named nurse concept.* Nursing Standard Jan 15 1992 Vol. 6. No. 17: 16-18.

Kron T 1991 The Management of Patient Care. 5th edition. W B Saunders, Philadelphia.

Manthey M 1980 The Practice of Primary Nursing. Blackwell, Oxford.

Tingle J H 1992 *Legal implications of standard setting.* British Journal of Nursing Vol. 1 No. 14: 728-31.

Wright S *The named nurse – A question of accountability.* Nursing Times March 11, 1992. Vol. 88. No. 11: 27-29.

3 Centrally Organised Methods of Quality Assurance

Introduction

In Chapter One some of the methods for implementing quality assurance in nursing were described briefly. It was stated that the implementation of quality assurance could be either centrally or locally organised and some of the main features of these two methods were noted. These have also been described as the traditional approach and the practitioner-based approach (Figure 1.3.1). The most noticeable difference between the two methods for the practising nurse at ward level is that centralised implementation is usually "done to", and locally organised implementation is "done by''. In the one case an assessment may have taken place in which the practitioner has played no part, while in the other, she is involved in the whole process. In this chapter we will look at the centralised method of implementing quality assurance.

Learning Outcomes

After studying this chapter the reader should be able to:
- explain how the term audit can be applied to health care;
- describe the main features of centrally organised methods of quality assurance;
- identify the strengths and weaknesses of centrally organised methods;
- compare and contrast traditional and practitioner-based approaches to quality assurance;
- describe how a centrally organised method of quality assurance may be introduced into a health care setting.

Nursing Audit

The word "audit" comes from the Latin word "auditus", "a hearing". It originally meant the hearing of facts and arguments about a situation to determine the truth. As the English language evolved the word in time lost its original broader meaning and became specifically concerned with the checking and endorsing of financial accounts. Today we think of an audit in these terms.

When used in connection with nursing, however, "audit" retains the old meaning. It involves supervising or "exercising assurance" on the quality of nursing care as it is carried out. A predetermined list of questions about the quality of care is

Traditional Quality Assurance Features	Practitioner-based Quality Assurance Features
standards and criteria generated by experts often at national level	standards and criteria generated and applied by practitioners to evaluate their own practice
measurement tools tested for validity and reliability	measurement tools devised at local level for topic-specific standards
external assessment of practitioners	peer assessment, self-assessment
practitioners expected to respond to recommendations for improvement	practitioners initiate recommendations for quality improvement
controlled externally, away from point of service delivery	owned and controlled by practitioners at point of service delivery, the patient has a central role
focus primarily on the process of care and inspecting the technical competence of practitioners	focus on identifying opportunities for improvement, rather than trying to eliminate poor quality
Examples: Monitor, Qualpacs, King's Fund Organisational Audit, Phaneuf's Audit	Examples: The unit-based approach, DySSSy

Figure 1.3.1 *Features of Traditional and Practitioner-based Approaches*

applied to the records of the care that has been delivered. The measurement usually takes place after the cycle of care has been completed and it is therefore normally retrospective. Traditionally, nursing audit is one of the centrally organised methods. It involves an investigation into data which has been recorded by nurses, the objectives being:
– to measure nursing performance in practice
– to assess nursing performance for reliability
– to make a statement about the quality of nursing performance in practice
– to improve, if necessary, future performance.

McGuire (1968) dates the beginning of medical audit in the USA back to the early 1900s. Nursing audit tools followed in the mid-1950s (Fisher, 1957), the majority of the early ones being retrospective, i.e. after the cycle of care has taken place and sometimes even after the discharge of the patient.

Until the mid-1980s, the term "audit" was synonymous with prescribed and published audits written by a few experts, which had been well researched for validity and reliability and were centrally organised. The three most commonly used at that time, particularly in the USA, were Phaneuf's Audit, Qualpacs and Rush Medicus Index. These have subsequently been adapted for use in the United Kingdom. In one instance Qualpacs and Phaneuf's Audit have been integrated and adapted to form one tool, the P.A. Measurement Scale. Likewise, Monitor, an adaptation of the Rush Medicus Index, has been widely used throughout the United Kingdom, and a proliferation of such tools has ensued with varying validity and reliability. Harvey (1987) reports that uptake of Monitor in English Health Authorities was 35.7%; unspecified audits, 17.9% and Qualpacs, 3.6%. A brief description of a number of these methods will be given, identifying some of the advantages and disadvantages in their use, and highlighting experiences.

Nursing audit, when carried out retrospectively, is based on a system which examines patient documentation of nursing care and draws conclusions about nursing performance based on these records. For such an audit to be successful, nursing documentation must be unambiguous and must be used and interpreted by every nurse in the same manner. For use in quality measurement nursing records should be regularly and systematically maintained so that the necessary information can be easily accessed and retrieved when required. Traditionally, this kind of nursing audit has been carried out by nurses who have not been directly involved with the patient, and is normally undertaken by staff of one service only, i.e. it is a uniprofessional approach.

It may be useful to consider here how some of these centrally organised methods have been constructed and implemented to help gain knowledge and expertise in methods of assuring quality. One of the most familiar audit tools is the technique developed in the United States by Maria Phaneuf, which she describes as: "a systematic, formal, and written appraisal, by nurses, of the content and process of nursing service from care records for discharged patients." (1964)

Phaneuf's Audit

In order to measure nursing performance, nursing activity is divided into the seven functions of nursing which were developed by Lesnik and Anderson in 1955. These functions are:
– the application and execution of the doctor's legal orders
– the observation of symptoms and reactions
– supervision of the patients
– supervision of those involved in care (with the exception of the physician)
– oral and written reporting and recording
– the application of techniques and nursing procedures
– the promotion of health through advice, direction and education.

Based on these seven functions, Phaneuf (1976) devised a total of 50 components to be applied to nursing performance, stated in terms of actions by nurses in relation to the patient, and in questions to be answered by the auditors as they review the patients' records. In this way the quality of nursing can be audited.

Every function is allocated a number of points. The scoring is based on a choice of one of three assessments for each component. For example, for Function 1, the values are as follows:
– yes (Y) = 7 points
– no (N) = 0 points
– uncertain (U) = 3 points.

There are six components applied to the first function from the Lesnik and Anderson list, giving a possible maximum of 42 points for the application and execution of the legal prescriptions of the doctor (Figure1.3.2).

	Yes	No	Uncertain	Totals
1. Medical diagnosis complete	7	0	3	
2. Prescriptions complete	7	0	3	
3. Prescriptions current	7	0	3	
4. Prescriptions promptly executed	7	0	3	
5. Evidence that nurse understood cause and effect	7	0	3	
6. Evidence that nurse took health history into account	7	0	3	
(42) Totals		0		

Figure 1.3.2 *Application and Execution of Legal Medical Prescriptions*

The values given to the assessment of the components of each function vary according to the importance of the function. In addition, the number of components allocated to each function also varies. Thus, for Function 4, Supervision of Those Participating in Care, there are only 4 components with the following values (Figure 1.3.3):
– yes = 5 points
– no = 0 points
– uncertain = 2 points.

The maximum total score for all of the seven functions is 200. The method of evaluation of the final score has been stipulated by Phaneuf as follows:
– 161-200 = excellent
– 121-160 = good
– 81-120 = incomplete
– 41-80 = poor
– 0-40 = unsafe

	Yes	No	Uncertain	Totals
1. Care taught to patient, family or others, nursing personnel	5	0	2	
2. Physical, emotional, mental capacity to learn considered	5	0	2	
3. Continuity of supervision to those taught	5	0	2	
4. Support of those giving care	5	0	2	
(20) Totals		0		

Figure 1.3.3 *Supervision of Those Participating in Care*

The implementation of such an approach involves the setting up of a nursing audit committee of at least five members. It is suggested that each member should review no more than ten patients each month, and that an auditor, when skilled, will take no more than 15 minutes to scrutinise a patient's record.

Phaneuf's Audit has been implemented extensively in the USA but has had limited application within the United Kingdom. It should be borne in mind that the seven functions of nursing were developed 40 years ago and the values given to these are now 20 years old. Although the method may now be dated, there are still lessons to be learned from its development and application as the basic processes continue to be relevant for today's practitioner. Phaneuf herself indicated that the method had certain limitations.

The first limitation is that the method has not been designed to measure care as it is taking place. The assessment always takes place retrospectively based on the nursing records, as a result of which it is only the recorded care, rather than the actual care, which can be the subject of assessment. In addition it is also possible that the actual care has been far more extensive than described, whereas the reverse might of course also be the case.

The second limitation indicated by Phaneuf is the fact that measurement does not revolve around the patient, but around the nursing record of the patient receiving care. To overcome these two limitations she recommends the implementation of a concurrent quality measurement tool from the patient's perspective as well as the retrospective audit of records. One of the widely used methods of measuring this is the Quality Patient Care Scale (QUALPACS) (Wandelt and Ager, 1974). This was derived from an earlier tool called the Slater Nursing Competencies Rating Scale (Slater, 1967; Wandelt and Stewart, 1975). Phaneuf recommends that this should complement the method that she has developed.

The third limitation she mentions is that although the audit can improve nursing report writing, this should not become the objective. In practice, Phaneuf's cautionary note about this last limitation is not always heeded. Thus Schroeder (1991) describes the phenomenon of report writing which is "socially desirable": nurses who know that nursing records are used for measuring quality make the effort to "improve" on their writing of reports.They record information which will meet the criteria and often ignore the reality of the actual care which has been delivered. In this way "socially desirable" reporting might emerge, which will, in the long run, have little to do with the actual nursing which has occurred.

> **Study Activity 1.**
> Are there occasions where you have identified differences between the care as it is described in the patient's nursing record, and care as it has been given? Consider the differences and write down your findings.

More Recent Developments

In the United Kingdom audit is a general term used to describe a mechanism for assessing and improving quality by promoting discussion among colleagues about care based on a review of nursing practice compared against preset criteria and standards. It would seem therefore, that the current working definition of audit is wider than a retrospective examination of the records and is increasingly embracing other methods of gathering information. Audit was originally a uniprofessional approach with medical and nursing staff working independently of each other but more recently, strategies and structures have been developed which have encouraged the establishment of clinical audit. Audit committees are usually set up in hospitals to consider the protocols proposed by practitioners wishing to implement specific audits, to control funding, to co-ordinate audit activity and to review particular topics. The main activities of any audit exercise are to find out what is actually happening, define what ought to be happening (i.e. set criteria and standards), compare observed practice with the standard, and implement any changes which are judged to be necessary.

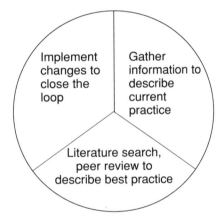

Figure 1.3.4 *Audit Cycle*

The audit process, often described as the *audit cycle*, is presented in Figure 1.3.4 (see also Figure 1.1.4, The Quality Assurance Cycle). Experience has shown that the difference between them, in broad terms, is that the standard setting experience focuses more immediately on the identification and implementation of desirable practice, and is therefore more easily seen as a quality improvement activity. On the other hand, although audit has been defined as a vehicle for change (and indeed, best practice has been achieved where it has been fully implemented), it may be perceived more immediately as a long look at current practice through the gathering of data which is then analysed, *probably* evaluated and *possibly* acted upon to promote change. To emphasise this point, a popular phrase, used particularly by our medical colleagues where audit activity is being carried out, is "We haven't yet closed the loop!" - in other words, the changes which have been recommended have yet to be made.

Monitor

Monitor, developed as part of the North West Staffing Levels Project (Goldstone et al, 1983), is the UK adaptation of the Rush Medicus Index which was devised in the United States in 1974 by Hegyvary, Haussmann, Jelinek and Newman. This is one of the most widely used and thoroughly tested methodologies in the USA.

Monitor is a centrally organised method of quality assurance which looks at the process of nursing care along with management of the ward and the environment. It is an indicator of nursing quality based on information gathered periodically at ward level. It is based on the nursing process and can be applied concurrently.

Monitor assesses the quality of nursing in relation to the following areas of care:
– planning and assessment
– physical care
– non-physical care
– evaluation of care.

The patients in a ward are classified according to categories of dependency, ranging from Category 1 – requiring minimal nursing care, to Category 4 - requiring intensive nursing care. Three patients are then randomly selected from each category and their care is scored either from observation, checking the nursing records, or talking with patients or nurses. Following data collection, the assessors score the results on a percentage basis, write a report, feed back results to staff at ward level and agree action plans. The assessors are usually senior clinical nurses who do not assess in those areas which are their direct managerial responsibility.

Monitor does not include all aspects of quality in nursing care and focuses on process rather than structure or outcome. A number of versions of Monitor have been developed covering various care groups, including community care, mental health, elderly care and nursing homes .

Implementation of this method has been found to be labour-intensive, particularly because a large amount of data is obtained through observation. Consequently this requires a great deal of preparation for the observers/assessors with regard to communication skills and observation techniques. It is particularly important that all observers know precisely what and how they should observe in order to maintain a high level of inter-rater reliability. In its implementation Monitor also requires that the observers have expertise in nursing.

Monitor can give an indication of nursing quality but this in itself is not sufficient to assume that points identified as weaknesses will automatically be improved. In this situation, in common with other centrally organised methods of quality assurance, these weaknesses will first have to be recognised and acknowledged as such by ward personnel before a change can be made.

The strengths and weaknesses of Monitor are shown in Figure 1.3.5.

Figure 1.3.5 *Advantages and Disadvantages of Monitor*

Advantages:
– an overview of quality is given
– both patient care and the environment where care takes place are examined
– the results produced are easily understood.

Disadvantages:
– a team of trained observers is needed
– staff have no involvement in the development of the criteria
– it may be misused to draw a false comparison between differing health care settings
– it may miss important key quality indicators
– a large amount of data is produced.

Qualpacs

The Quality of Patient Care Scale, or Qualpacs (op cit), was derived from the Slater Nursing Competencies Scale (op cit) which was designed to measure the quality of individual nurse performance. Items from the Slater Scale which assess individual performance have been reworded to shift the emphasis from nurse to patient.

Qualpacs organised nursing activities into 68 elements of care which have been classified under the following six broad headings:

1. *Psychosocial: Individual*
   actions directed towards meeting psychosocial needs of
   individual patients   15 items
2. *Psychosocial : Group*
   meeting needs as members of a group   8 items
3. *Physical*
   actions directed towards meeting the physical needs
   of patients   15 items
4. *General*
   actions directed towards either psychosocial or physical   15 items
5. *Communication*
   communication on behalf of the patient   8 items
6. *Professional implications*
   care given which reflects initiative and responsibility
   indicative of professional expectations   7 items

Qualpacs is a measure of nursing process and the data is usually collected concurrently by direct observation. Observation is carried out by a minimum of two trained observers to reduce all risk of observer bias. Usually five patients or 15%, whichever is higher, is the target group and care is observed over a two-hour period. More realistic findings may be obtained if assessments take place at various times of the day and night.

Permission of patients should always be sought in advance. Assessors receive a verbal report on the patients selected, they consult patient documentation, then they develop their care plan of what they expect to see. For observation to be complete, observers need permission to enter behind screens.

During observation, all nurse–patient interactions are broken down and allocated to one or more of the 68 items. Each item is then rated on a five-point scale, with the fixed standard being the care expected from a first-level registered nurse. After the observation period is completed indirect evidence is collected from patient documentation. The mean scores for each item are added together then divided by the number of observations.

Figure 1.3.6 *Advantages and Disadvantages of Qualpacs*

Advantages
– rigorously tested for validity and reliability
– since actual care is being observed the results are more accurate than judging care from patient documentation.

Disadvantages
– values are American
– requires highly skilled and trained observers
– time-consuming
– observer bias
– criticised for being subjective and reliant on professional judgement
– scoring system is complicated
– it gives a narrow dimension of quality with the emphasis on psychosocial and communicative aspects of care
– invasion of privacy.

Study Activity 2.
Make a list of the different dimensions of quality that are being measured in the three methods outlined above.

Conclusion

The centrally organised methods of applying quality assurance demonstrate in a relatively short period of time the strengths and weaknesses of nursing care provided, in relation to the level of quality being considered within the instrument. It is then the responsibility of the staff in the clinical area to ensure that these findings are put to the best possible use, i.e. to maintain the strengths and to improve on the weaknesses.

Attempts have been made to establish correlation between quality assessments using different tools. Giovannetti et al (1986) examined the Rush Medicus Index, an outcome audit tool and a chart audit. Their findings were that there was little correlation among them, suggesting that different dimensions of quality were being measured. Other studies have been unable to establish correlations between Qualpacs and the Rush Medicus Index and Phaneuf's Audit (Ventura, 1980; Ventura et al, 1982).

Study Activity 3.

Find out if the area you are working in or where you are a student has been involved in any quality assurance activity similar to those described in this chapter.

a. What form did the exercise take?

b. Were the criteria predetermined?

c. Who carried out the exercise?

d. How were the results fed back to staff?

One of the features of the centrally organised methods is that the nurses who provide the patient with immediate care often have only limited involvement in the assessment process. Taking note of the results on its own will not help to motivate them to devise and implement a change of plan, especially if the findings indicate a weakness in the clinical area which they may not recognise as such. In order to accomplish change, the staff concerned have to admit to the need for it and should be able to identify the improvements which are needed, so that afterwards it is obvious that change was necessary. If this is not the case, resistance to the change may occur and in the long run quality assurance itself might be regarded as a threat.

Harvey (1991) in her evaluation of approaches to assessing quality of nursing care found that "the process of implementing a quality assurance tool is more important than the tool itself. It is suggested that a bottom-up approach to implementation…is seen to result in more favourable staff responses and positive programme outcomes". In the next chapter we go on to consider a bottom-up approach to quality assurance where the criteria and standards are determined by the practitioner.

Study Activity 4.

Changing practice is not always easy to accomplish. Discuss factors that would motivate you to change your practice.

References

Fisher P R 1957 *The nursing audit.* Nursing Outlook 5:10 590-592.

Giovannetti P B, Kerr J C, Bay K and Buchan J 1986 Measuring Quality of Nursing Care: Analysis and Validity of Selected Instruments. Final report of research project. University of Alberta, Alberta.

Goldstone L A, Ball J A, Collier M M 1983 Monitor. An Index of the Quality of Nursing Care for Acute Medical and Surgical Wards (North West Staffing Levels Project) Newcastle upon Tyne Polytechnic Projects, Newcastle upon Tyne.

Harvey G 1987 *Compiling a directory.* Nursing Times Vol. 83 No. 44: 49-50

Harvey G 1991 *An evaluation of approaches to assessing the quality of nursing care using (predetermined) quality assurance tools.* Journal of Advanced Nursing 16: 277-286.

Jelinek R C, Haussmann R K D, Hegyvary S T and Newman J F 1974. A Methodology for Monitoring Quality of Nursing Care. US Department of Health, Education and Welfare, DHEW Publication No. (HRA) 74-25.

Lesnik M J and Anderson B E 1955 Nursing Practice and the Laboratory. Lippincott, Philadelphia.

McGuire R L 1968 *Bedside nursing audit.* American Journal of Nursing, 68:10 2146-2148

Phaneuf M C 1964 *A nursing audit method. Appraisal of patient care from the records of service can be developed by nurses into a specific method of audit.* Nursing Outlook, 12(5): 42-45.

Phaneuf M C 1976 The Nursing Audit – Self-regulation in Nursing Practice. Appleton-Century-Crofts, New York.

Schroeder P 1991 The Encyclopedia of Nursing Care Quality. Aspen Publishers, Gaithersberg, MD.

Slater D 1967 The Slater Nursing Competencies Scale. College of Nursing, Wayne State University, Detroit.

Wandelt M A, Ager J W 1974 The Slater Nursing Competencies Rating Scale. Appleton-Century-Crofts, New York.

Ventura M R, Hageman P T, Slakter M J, Fox R N 1982 *Correlation of two quality nursing care measures.* Research in Nursing and Health 5: 37-43.

Ventura M R 1980 *Correlation between the quality patient care scale and the Phaneuf audit.* International Journal of Nursing Studies 17: 155-62.

Further Reading

Fox R N and Ventura M R 1984 *Internal psychometric characteristics of the Quality Patient Care Scale.* Nursing Research 24 (1): 112-117.

Giebing H A 1987 *Unit-based approach for nursing quality assurance in the Netherlands: one year experience.* Australian Clinical Review, 7 (24): 28-31.

Harvey G 1988 *The right tools for the job.* Nursing Times, Vol. 84 No. 26: 47-49.

Harvey G 1988 *More tools for the job.* Nursing Times, Vol. 84 No. 28: 33-34.

Hegyvary S T and Haussmann R K D 1976 *Monitoring nursing care quality.* Journal of Nursing Administration, 6(9): 3-9.

Trussel P M and Strand N A 1978 *A comparison of concurrent and retrospective audits of the same patients.* Journal of Nursing Administration, 8(5): 33-38.

Willis L D and Linwood M E (eds) 1984 Measuring the Quality of Care. Churchill Livingstone, Edinburgh.

4 Locally Organised Methods of Quality Assurance

Introduction

In Chapter Three we described some of the features of centrally organised quality assurance and discussed some of the experiences which have been encountered in utilising this approach. Some of the limitations of this method were pointed out, two of the more important ones being:
- the lack of a well-defined link between the identification of need for change and the accomplishment of the measures to bring about improvement
- the lack of involvement of the nursing staff in the audit itself, which may lead to a feeling of resentment towards, and estrangement from the audit and its results.

This chapter describes the locally organised approach to quality assurance. This method can be applied retrospectively, concurrently or prospectively.

Learning Outcomes

After studying this chapter the reader should be able to:
- describe the early standards of care work;
- list and explain the six principles on which DySSSy is based;
- describe the three phases of the quality assurance cycle;
- outline the four steps in the describing phase;
- outline the four steps in the auditing phase;
- outline the five steps in the taking action phase;
- describe how practitioner-based quality assurance can be introduced into a health-care setting;
- describe how groups are organised to create an effective support structure;
- identify the advantages and disadvantages of locally organised methods of quality assurance.

Dynamic Standard Setting System (DySSSy)

The most widely recognised locally organised method is the Dynamic Standard Setting System (RCN, 1990) or an adaptation of it. This system is now known as the Dynamic Quality Improvement programme (DQI) but in this text we will use the abbreviation DySSSy.

In health-care settings where this system has been implemented successfully, firm foundations for the subsequent development of a total quality management approach have been established. This successful implementation has been due in particular to the total involvement of people within the organisation taking responsibility for improvement through projects of manageable proportions for which they have ownership. Where the system has been less helpful is in achieving commitment from the "top" of the organisation, a necessary component of a total quality management approach. This vital ingredient has not always been evident in supporting DySSSy projects due to a number of reasons, one being that it may be perceived as time-consuming. Experience has shown, however, that DySSSy in its implementation integrates the change process with quality assurance principles and therefore does take some time.

Beginnings

Much of the work on developing nursing quality assurance systems in the United Kingdom has been based on the professional activity of the Royal College of Nursing (RCN). The RCN's commitment to standards of care and promoting excellence in nursing practice has spanned almost three decades of work. This commenced in 1965 with the first *Standards of Nursing Care Project* headed by Baroness Jean McFarlane (1970), and was followed by the work of an expert group set up in 1978 under the chairmanship of Dame Sheila Quinn, the then President of the RCN (RCN, 1980, 1981; WHO, 1982, 1984). The present developments have grown from this earlier work, and the setting up of the *RCN Standards of Care Project* in 1985 started the third phase of activity (RCN, 1989). It was in this third phase that the Dynamic Standard Setting System was initiated. Much of the work in its early development was undertaken by Helen Kendall (1986, 1988).

Principles

The Dynamic Standard Setting System is a programme for setting, monitoring and evaluating standards of nursing practice at ward level. It adopts a problem-solving, patient-focused approach to continuous quality improvement and has been developed from a number of primary sources as follows:
– Lang's quality assurance cycle (1976)
– Donabedian's description of structure, process and outcome (1966)
– the work on standards of the Manitoba Association of Registered Nurses (MARN) (Scherer, 1985)
– Schroeder and Maibusch's unit-based approach (1984).

The underlying philosophy of this system is that the judgements and actions of "ordinary practitioners" should determine the quality of care provided. This is in contrast to the more traditional approach of evaluating quality by making a comparison of preformulated expert standards with actual practice. In support of this approach Donabedian suggests that standards can be described on the basis of how they are derived, *normatively* or *empirically*. Normative standards are "expert" standards concerning what ought to be done. Empirically derived standards, on the other hand, represent what is actually done.

DySSSy is based on six key principles:

- *owned and controlled by practitioners*
  DySSSy is a system which is "done by" rather than "done to" those carrying out nursing care. Practitioners are more closely involved in the activity than in other systems and they have a degree of control throughout the entire process. This includes control over the subject or activity chosen, the improvements to be achieved and the ongoing monitoring method. Thus the process is seen as relevant, it is valued and there is more likelihood of commitment to the improvement.
  The term "ownership" has sometimes been misunderstood at the introduction of quality assurance activities. It does not necessarily mean starting from the beginning or reinventing the wheel when developing a new standard, but rather using an existing standard and adopting or adapting the standard for one's own client group and area of work.

- *participation and involvement of practitioners*
  The "done by" aspect encourages the whole team at local level to be more actively involved in the process, including monitoring and evaluating their standards.

- *patient/client focused*
  The primary objective of the activity is to describe quality interventions in terms of the impact on the patient, the patient's experiences and any health gain. This involves outcome evaluation as well as the identification of structure and process variables related to care.

- *situation-based*
  Standards and criteria are developed with sensitivity to the care group, the environment and the organisation's philosophy of care. This enables the standard to have a high degree of relevance to the setting where care is taking place.

- *set within achievability*
  The emphasis is on achievability rather than minimum, ideal or optimum standards.This reflects and reinforces other important features of the system, notably that standard setting is both a dynamic and a realistic pursuit. It is worth while noting that achievability is not enough on its own, and desirability must also be a consideration.

- *interprofessional potential*
  In order to provide a comprehensive and quality service interprofessional activity is required. By taking a patient centred approach, standards can be developed by interprofessional teams using DySSSy's principles and techniques.

Study Activity 1.
Take any three of the six principles on which DySSSy is based. Relate these to any quality assurance activity which has already taken place in your clinical area. Discuss in your group how these principles were applied to the activity.

Implementing DySSSY

DySSSy is used extensively by nurses and other health-care staff throughout the United Kingdom. The starting-point has to be with practitioners. The system does not require that you start out with a set of preformulated standards. This "bottom-up" philosophy enables practitioners to address issues of quality within their own area of work. It is also important, however, that support for the whole system comes from the top of the organisation.

A group of practitioners form a standard setting group to work through the steps of the quality assurance cycle. Throughout the standard setting process, the group should work with a trained facilitator (see also Chapter 5). The initial implementation of the DySSSy system is very much a learning process, both for practitioners and facilitators, enabling the development of evaluation skills for practice.

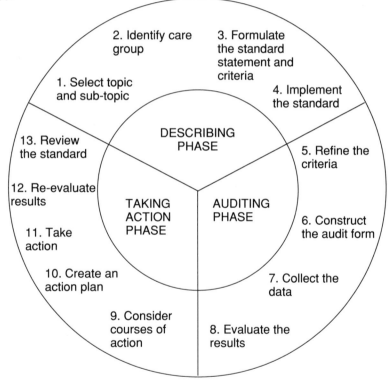

Figure 1.4.1 *The Quality Assurance Cycle (Adapted from Quality Patient Care, RCN, 1990)*

A. The Describing Phase

In this phase the standard and criteria are established by identifying and agreeing on elements of good practice. Whether a nursing situation is "good", "bad", "desirable" or "undesirable" is determined by the nursing values which influence day-to-day practice. An example of this is the perceptible shift in nursing values away from medical values and the medical model. Traditionally, within medical care, and therefore nursing care, success was measured by physical cure, whereas in current practice the caring aspects of nursing have come to play the major role. Successful nursing in today's world may well be about helping the patient and family to cope with a physical disability or indeed a peaceful and pain-free death.

Scientific knowledge also affects nursing values. Consider, for instance, the impact which technological and scientific developments have on nursing practice in the areas of care delivery and the equipment which is used.

Other important values can be identified from the patient's perspective. These may include:
– the safety of the patient and his environment
– the degree to which individualised nursing care is systematically provided
– continuity in nursing care
– self-motivation in the recovery process
– patient involvement in the planning of nursing care and in decision-making
– privacy
– confidentiality of data
– health promotion and education.

Nursing staff may regard the following areas as being equally important:
– safety in professional practice
– statutory requirements and competencies
– organisation of work
– education
– in-service training/refresher courses
– research
– professional accountability
– working environment
– communication and collaboration with other health-care providers.

As the standard is developed the nursing values which affect the activity chosen are agreed and may be made explicit. It is more likely, however, that at this early stage the discussion is around the more tangible and observable activities which would be carried out as a result of what is valued.

1. Select a Topic and Sub-topic
It is useful to identify a topic and sub-topic (see below) so that the standard can be focused, categorised and subsequently catalogued or indexed. For example, a group on a surgical ward may wish to improve the quality of pain relief given to patients (see Figure 1.4.4). The response to pain is a very subjective and personal experience and, therefore, using the topic list illustrated in Figure 1.4.2, the subject of pain relief could be categorised under the topic of individualised care, with the sub-topic being pain relief. To take another example, a communication problem between hospital and community nursing staff on discharge arrangements might be identified under the topic *continuity of care*, and the sub-topic *discharge planning*.

Standards of Nursing Care Topic List	
	Code
Individualised Care	01
Continuity of Care	02
Independence and Involvement	03
Privacy	04
Safety	05
Confidentiality	06
Health Education	07
Patients'/Clients'/Residents' Rights	08
Therapeutic Environment	09
Personnel	10
Statutory Nurse/Midwife Education	11
Continuing Education for Nurses/Midwives	12
Research	13
Professional Accountability	14
Management	15
Midwife Supervision	16

Figure 1.4.2 *The Topic List*

Although it would be "tidier" and perhaps logical to identify the topic and sub-topic at this early stage, it is often the case that the topic and sub-topic only become clear or more evident during the course of developing the standard. Effective facilitation, especially active listening, helps to focus, refocus and identify the topic and sub-topic. More often than not, the standard setting process begins with the identification of a specific issue or activity which is of concern to nurses and/or patients. The group then works from the specific (sub-topic) to the general (topic).

The subject or activity which the group chooses will usually be an area which is in need of improvement, or an area of concern which may be perceived as a problem. However, it could equally be an area of particular interest, or an innovative idea which needs to be checked out in practice. The standards and criteria will be influenced by the values and beliefs of the practitioners involved and these will be made more explicit during the process of agreeing the standard.

In a hospital context, data originating from complaints, centralised audit activity or specialist nurses (for example, tissue viability, control of infection) can all serve as a source of inspiration for subject choice. In a community context, themes like terminal care, pressure sore prevention and treatment, and continuity of care are issues frequently addressed. It is important that nurses within a primary health-care team or department are in agreement about the choice of subject and are willing to give it their support. To facilitate this the following questions might be asked:
– How frequently does the problem arise?
– What impact does it have on quality?
– Can it lead to patient discomfort, or even fatal error?

54

– Can the problem be solved within the ward or base?
– Does the ward have the human resources to achieve an improvement?

2. Identify the Care Group

As well as defining the topic and sub-topic, the standard setting group identifies the care group for which the standard is applicable. The choice of care group will of course affect how the standard is constructed. For example, discharge planning for the elderly client group would require different criteria from a discharge plan for babies in a special care baby unit. In the example of the standard for pain relief in a surgical ward, the care group might be, for instance, patients undergoing major abdominal surgery.

> **Study Activity 2.**
> List four areas of nursing practice in the clinical setting with which you are most familiar that need to be improved.

3. Formulate the Standard Statement and Criteria

Standards are general statements, and criteria are descriptive elements of these. The broad objective of the standard is outlined in the form of a statement specifying a level of quality. In the example referred to earlier, this might be: *Analgesia is given to meet individual need and promote recovery.* Such a standard is formulated on the basis of established values. The criteria are items or variables selected as indicators of whether or not the standard is being achieved. The criteria render the components of the standard "visible", as it were, and they are also the gauge by which quality can be measured. They are detailed indicators, finely tuned for a particular client group in a particular setting. These criteria need to be:

R elevant
U nderstandable
M easurable
B ehavioural
A chievable

> **Study Activity 3.**
> Take one of the areas for improvement which you have identified in Study Activity 2:
> **a.** Describe how that activity is being carried out at present.
> **b.** Consider why it is being done in that particular way.
> **c.** Suggest how that activity *should* be carried out.

Three types of criteria are identified (Figure 1.4.3)

Structure criteria
These describe resources in the system which are necessary for the successful completion of the activity under review - in other words, the people and things required. *Who and what are needed? Which resources should be available?*

Figure 1.4.3 *Model Layout*

Standard Reg. No.	
Topic	(Main heading chosen from Nursing Standards Index)
Sub-Topic	(States the specific aspects of the topic covered by this standard)
Care Group	(Makes the standard specific to a particular setting and applicable to a group of patients)
Source of Production	(Area to which authors belong)
Standard Statement	(This describes the desired outcome of nursing care; states an expectation of the quality of care or level of service)

Achieve Standard By (A commitment to achieve the standard within the setting and within a specified time)

Review Standard By (Periodic review to ensure that the content remains acceptable)

Signature of Responsible Nurse

Date

STRUCTURE	PROCESS	OUTCOME
(What must be provided in order to achieve the standard)	(Follows the framework of the nursing process)	(Describes the effect of the nursing care/the achievement)

Physical environment
Equipment
Staff numbers
  Skill level
  Knowledge
Information
Organisational system
	The nurse assesses…
	The nurse includes in the plan…
	The nurse does
	The nurse reviews
		The patient is…
		The patient does…
		The patient receives…
		Measurable indicators…
		Observable behaviours…

Process criteria
These relate to actions undertaken by staff in order to achieve certain results, including assessment techniques, intervention patterns, patient education or information-giving - in other words, what needs to be done and by whom. *How should the action be carried out? Who will do it?*

Outcome criteria
These describe the desired effect of nursing care in terms of patient behaviours, levels of knowledge, patient satisfaction, statistical indicators, health status or quality of life. *What should be the result of the action?*

The formulation of structure, process and outcome criteria makes it possible to give a picture of the desired quality (Figure 1.4.4). Obviously the set standards and criteria will always have to fit in with the aims of the organisation and existing statutes governing professional conduct. In formulating standards and criteria, reference can be made to nursing literature and research, already established standards and criteria and one's own experience and knowledge.

> **Study Activity 4.**
> Take the area for improvement you have chosen in Study Activity 3. Refer also to Figure 1.4.3 (Model Layout for a Standard).
> **a.** Identify broad desirable aims for the area of improvement.
> **b.** From these aims formulate your standard statement.
> **c.** Choose a topic from Figure 1.4.2 and identify a sub-topic.
> **d.** Identify the care group.
> **e.** Using your answer to Study Activity 3c, select items which can be refined into structure, process and outcome criteria.
> **f.** Formulate a minimum of three each for structure, process and outcome criteria.

4. Implement the Standard
Using the structure-process-outcome framework, practitioners break down the subject area to identify criteria which they see as key to the provision of a good standard of care. In order to reflect the dynamic nature of the standard, the group specify "implement by", "achieve by" dates (Figure 1.4.4) in order to set a realistic timescale for accomplishing the necessary changes in practice.

The criteria which are established form the basis of an action plan and subsequent audit activity. At this point the standard setting group will go on to do one of two things. If the priority is an urgent and immediate need for improvement then the standard is implemented, i.e. the agreed action is carried out. If, on the other hand, further information is needed to identify the cause and the extent of the problem, then current practice may need to be carefully scrutinised. In this case an audit is required before making any changes.

Figure 1.4.4 *Standard for Analgesia*

Standard Reg. No.	01/116		Achieve Standard By 31/01/88
Topic	Individualised care		Review Standard By 01/02/93
Sub-Topic	Administration of analgesia following abdominal surgery		Signature of DNS
Care Group	Surgical patients in hospital		Signature of Senior Nurse
Source of Production	Surgical unit		Date 26/10/87
Standard Statement	All patients receive post-operative analgesia to meet individual needs and promote recovery		

STRUCTURE	PROCESS	OUTCOME
Code of practice for medicines is available in ward.	The nurse observes, assesses and reports individual patient's condition and response to pain.	The patient expresses that pain is controlled.
There is a written medicine policy.	The nurse records findings in appropriate documentation.	The degree of pain and site are identified.
The nurse has a knowledge of analgesia and contraindications.	The nurse assesses in consultation with anaesthetist, consultant and doctor.	Analgesia is given by prescribed route.
The nurse is aware of the various routes of administration: i.e. oral, P.R., I.M., I.V. syringe driver, epidural and blocks. Ward protocol identifying expected response times.	The nurse administers the correct medication as prescribed.	Problems highlighted are recorded, evaluated and resolved.
Each patient has correct, current prescription sheet to provide 24-hour pain relief.	The nurse records accurately the route and drug administered in nursing notes.	The patient is relaxed and able to be moved freely.
Formal communication exists among all members of the care team.	The nurse evaluates the effectiveness of analgesia given and informs doctor if pain is not relieved within response time specified for routes of administration.	The patient is able to participate in activities of living/treatment, e.g. physiotherapy.
	The nurse documents reasons of pain not being controlled, i.e. haemorrhage, shock, temperature.	Post-operative complications are lessened.
		The patient is not afraid of further surgery if required.

B. The Auditing Phase

After writing the standard, the group devises a way of auditing; that is, checking out whether or not they are achieving the levels of care they have specified in their standard.

5. Refine the Criteria

By making use of RUMBA, practitioners check the content, structure and order of their criteria. It could be argued that this stage could equally be part of the describing phase.

6. Construct the Audit Form/Protocol

An audit form or protocol is devised from the completed standard and the following questions are considered:

WHAT needs to be examined? Some or all of the criteria are turned into questions to check how well the standard is being met. This data must be relevant to the formulated criteria.

WHO should collect the information?

HOW should it be collected (e.g. by asking the patient or nurse, or by observation or checking records)? The data must be obtainable with a minimum amount of time, effort and disruption to the patient and the clinical area.

HOW OFTEN does information need to be collected to indicate whether or not the standard is being achieved? The time frame during which data is obtained must be agreed and specified beforehand.

WHEN is the best time to collect the data? The data should not be collected during a period of abnormal activity unless the context of the audit is specified.

HOW MANY patients, observations, responses need to be included to provide reliable information? This will depend on the number of times the activity takes place and the number of patients involved.

If the care group is a large one, for example all adult surgical patients, a large sample can be found fairly quickly. If, on the other hand, the care group is specialised, for example, patients with a particular condition, the time frame will need to be longer. If the frequency is unknown, hospital statistics can provide information on the frequency of such cases. Estimating sample size is complicated and it is vital that the sample is representative of what is usual. To avoid bias, random sampling of patients may be one method of accomplishing this, for example, selecting every third admission to the ward.

These questions can be applied to our pain management example as illustrated in Figure 1.4.5.

Study Activity 5.
Using the standard statement and the criteria you have developed in Study Activity 4, check these against the RUMBA items.

Figure 1.4.5 *Audit Form/Protocol*

AUDIT PROTOCOL

Audit Objective: To find out whether post-operative analgesia meets individual needs and promotes recovery.
Time Frame: One month June 1994
Sample: Every other patient – 3rd post-op day/all nursing staff/ 50% of records/1 observation weekly of environment.
Auditors: CN Smart (Theatres)
Date: 1/4/94

Target Group	Method	Code	Audit Criteria
Patients	Ask	01	Is the patient satisfied with his pain control?
		01	Ask the patient to describe his pain on a scale of 1-10.
		05	Can the patient move freely without suffering pain
		05a	a. in and out of bed?
		05b	b. during physiotherapy?
		05c	c. participating in activities of living?
		08	If further surgery is scheduled – can the patient state that he is not fearful of pain?
Patients	Observe	05	Does the patient show non-verbal signs of pain?
Nurses	Ask	S1	Can each nurse on duty outline the key points in the code of practice for medicines?
		S2	Can each nurse on duty outline the key points in the medicine policy?
		S3	Can each nurse on duty describe analgesia used and complications?
		S4	Can each nurse on duty describe common routes of administration of analgesia?
		S6	Can each nurse on duty describe how interprofessional communication takes place to ensure effective pain relief with
		S6a	a. medical staff?
		S6b	b. paramedical staff?
		S6c	c. others?
Records	Check	P1/P2	Has an assessment taken place which describes the patient's condition and response to pain?
		P1	If individual painometers are in use document levels identified in sample.
		P5	Does the record accurately identify route and medication administered?
		P6	Does the record indicate that an evaluation of the effectiveness of analgesia has taken place?
		P6/P7	Does the record indicate that further action has been taken when ineffective?
Environment	Observe	S1	Is the code of practice for medicines accessible on ward?
		S2	Is the medicine policy accessible on ward?
		S4	Is the protocol for response times to routes of administration accessible on ward?
		S5	Does each patient have a current, correct prescription sheet?

7. Collect the Data

Although an external auditor may be invited to participate in the assessment, control of the auditing exercise remains with the practitioners. For example, a staff nurse member of the standard setting group may be nominated as the auditor. However, as practitioners become more confident with the system and peer monitoring develops, the likelihood of an external auditor participating increases. This might be a quality assurance officer or a colleague from another profession. Where the auditor is a member of staff on the ward being audited, the advantages include greater sensitivity to the subject and the possibility of subsequent behaviour change taking place in that particular setting. The external auditor has the advantage of bringing objectivity to the situation and her non-involvement in the care setting gives more credibility to the results of the exercise. The data collected is recorded on the audit record (Figure 1.4.6) and analysed to compare the expected with the actual compliance.

The audit record may be in the form of a checklist which can be completed by the auditor after an action has been performed. This checklist can also be the starting-point for group discussion. Nurses can discuss their actions, checking them off against the items on the checklist. A checklist typically requires answers that can be given in terms of "yes" or "no", "done" or "not done", "present" or "not present". The category "not applicable" can also be used. This, however, should not be restricted to "yes" and "no" answers only, as descriptive findings can be documented as comments (Figure 1.4.6). As previously stated, the structured inquiry should be focused on the target groups as identified in Figure 1.4.5. The questions which are asked will have been carefully constructed beforehand and the completed checklist should give a genuine picture of actual practice.

Structured observation involves scrutiny of a number of prearranged aspects relating to the subject chosen. It should be agreed upon in advance how the observation is to be evaluated so that differences in observation and evaluation between observers can be avoided. For this stage to be effective, careful training is required to ensure inter-rater reliability.

8. Evaluate the Results

After completing the audit record, the auditor summarises the findings and presents these back to the group in the form of an audit summary (Figure 1.4.7). Using this summary, the group highlights discrepancies, discusses possible causes and draws conclusions in order to develop an action plan to address the problems identified from the audit. Practitioners need to consider the following questions in relation to the design of the standard and the audit form:
- Are the discrepancies due to poor design of the audit tool/instrument?
- Is the method of data collection inappropriate?
- Is the standard set unrealistic?

During this process it is possible to set a realistic norm/compliance rate for each criterion. This means that for each criterion an acceptable level may be determined. In some cases, a criterion will have to score fully (100%) for the quality to be judged acceptable, but in others it may be that a margin is allowed,

Figure 1.4.6 *Audit Record*

Audit Objective — To find out whether post-operative analgesia meets individual needs and promotes recovery.
PT/Carer Sample — Every other patient on 3rd Post-op day/50% records
Staff Sample — All trained staff on duty at time of audit
Ward/Env Sample — 1 observation weekly
Auditors — C N Smart
Time Frame — One month 1/6/94 to 30/6/94

Actual Sample — 20 patients/10 records/7 nurses
KEY
Y = Yes N = No
NA = Not Applicable NR = Non-Response
E = Expected A = Actual
Date 1/4/94

TARGET GROUP	CODE	OBSERVATIONS (Obs)										TOTALS			COMPLIANCE		COMMENTS
		1	2	3	4	5	6	7	8	9	10	Obs	Y	N	E	A	
Patients	O1	Y	Y	Y	Y	Y	N	N	N	N	N	20	14	6	100	70	No pain thermometer/chart in use
	O1	55	46	35	44	34	47	64	64	55	55	20	13	7	100	65	
	O5 a	Y	Y	Y	Y	Y	N	N	N	N	N	20	13	7	100	65	
	O5 b	Y	Y	Y	Y	Y	Y	N	N	N	N	20	12	8	100	60	
	O5 c	N	N	Y	Y	Y	N	N	Y	Y	Y				100	50	
	O8	–	N	Y	–	–	–	–	–	–	–	2	1	1	80	25	Only applicable to 2 Is this acceptable?
	O5	N	Y	N	N	N	Y	N	N	N	N	20	5	15			
Nurses	S1	Y	Y	Y	Y	Y	Y	N				7	6	1	100	86	
	S2	Y	Y	Y	Y	Y	Y	Y				7	7	0	100	100	Need for update on the importance of the specified code of practice and interprofessional communication with paramedical staff
	S3	Y	Y	Y	Y	Y	Y	N				7	6	1	100	86	
	S4	Y	Y	Y	Y	Y	Y	Y				7	7	0	100	100	
	S6 a	Y	Y	Y	Y	Y	Y	Y				7	7	0	100	100	
	S6 b	Y	Y	Y	Y	Y	Y	N				7	6	1	100	86	
	S6 c	No others identified															
Records	P1/P2	Y	Y	Y	N	N	N	N	Y	Y	Y	10	6	4	100	60	Find out how the assessment takes place.
	P1	Not applicable															
	P5	Y	Y	Y	Y	Y	Y	Y	Y	Y	Y	10	10	0	100	100	
	P6	Y	N	N	Y	Y	N	Y	N	Y	Y	10	6	4	100	60	Reinforce the importance of record keeping
	P6/P7	Y	Y	Y	Y	Y	N	N	N	NA	NA	8	4	4	100	50	
Environment	S1	Y	Y	Y	Y							4	4	0	100	100	Prescription sheet in theatre although patient 3 hours post-op. Is this unusual?
	S2	Y	Y	Y	Y							4	4	0	100	100	
	S4	Y	Y	Y	Y							4	4	0	100	100	
	S5	Y	Y	Y	N							4	3	1	100	75	

Figure 1.4.7 *Audit Summary*

Audit Objective	To find out whether post-operative analgesia meets individual needs and promotes recovery.
PT/Carer Sample	Every other patient on 3rd Post-op day/50% records
Staff Sample	All trained staff on duty at time of audit
Ward/Env Sample	1 observation weekly
Auditors	C N Smart
Time Frame	1/6/94 to 30/6/94 **Date**

ACTIVITY	FINDINGS	CONCLUSIONS
Professional knowledge and access to policies.	All information specified was accessible. 6 out of 7 nurses were able to state keypoints.	Updating required on code of practice.
Interprofessional communication.	One nurse was unable to describe communication system with paramedical staff.	Is this an isolated incident? Check communication systems in general with medical, nursing and paramedical staff.
Recording of assessment and management of pain.	Assessment describing condition and response to pain was documented in 60% of records. No pain thermometer or pain assessment chart was in use. Evaluation of effectiveness of pain relief was documented in 60% of records. Evaluation following ineffective pain relief was documented in 50% of records Current prescription sheets were present with one exception.	Patients' response to pain requires to be given a higher priority and documented accurately. More work is required on assessment and evaluation of pain relief. Second evaluation needs to be documented. Was the exception an isolated incident? Why did it happen? – an emergency occurred.
Patient mobility and recovery.	70% were satisfied with pain relief. 65% were able to move/be moved freely. 25% were not showing non-verbal signs of pain.	There is a need to investigate further why 35% of patients have restricted mobility – is this acceptable? Is it related to a particular care group? Relate these findings to the scale as identified by patients and to restricted mobility.

so that the quality may be judged acceptable when the score is, for example, 80%. Since standards are set within achievability, then a 100% rate seems a reasonable expectation.

> **Study Activity 6.**
> With the standard from Study Activity 4 as your main source of information, construct an audit form, identifying:
> **a.** *the objective of the audit* – this should reflect your standard statement;
> **b.** *the time frame* – how long the audit will last;
> **c.** *the sample* – ward environment, care group, documentation;
> **d.** *the auditor* – who will be responsible;
> **e.** *the audit criteria* – select some or all of the criteria in the standard;
> **f.** *the method and target group* – how the information is to be gathered and from whom.

The evaluation consists of a comparison between desirable performance and actual performance. In other words, the data about an actual performance is judged against the criteria which have been set for that performance. The scores should then be compared. It should be noted here that the comparison should not be made simply by the addition of all the scores, as some of the criteria may be of more significance than others and will therefore carry a higher value.

C. The Taking Action Phase
The next step is to consider conclusions and to identify areas where action is required.

9. Consider Courses of Action
Possible courses of action are discussed identifying those responsible for changes and setting realistic time-scales. These actions may include:
- reviewing the standard
- implementing the standard more thoroughly
- changing the method of data collection.

When there is a valid reason for an action not meeting its criteria, for example a reduction in staff numbers since the original action plan was conceived, then the criteria will have to be reviewed. In cases where actions fail to meet reasonable criteria, a plan for corrective action will have to be set up.

10. Create an Action Plan
An action plan for improvement is finalised and implemented (Figure 1.4.8). This may also include, for example, in-service training or continuing education, the development of a nursing care plan or assessment tool, or redesigning patient documentation to facilitate the gathering of relevant information. It is very

Figure 1.4.8 *Action Plan*

IDENTIFIED PROBLEM	SUGGESTED ACTION	MEMBER OF STAFF RESPONSIBLE	TIME PERIOD
Key staff members were unaware of detail in code of practice and the system for interprofessional communication.	Discuss with staff as individuals the importance of the documents identified and relate to personal accountability.	C.N. Swift	By 31.8.94
	Set up an afternoon session to discuss interprofessional communication (document system)	C.N. Swift Senior Physio Jones	By 30.9.94
Lack of documented evaluation of pain relief.	Set up sub-group to review current pain documentation.	S.N. Ross	By 30.11.94
Need for more detailed assessment of response to pain.	Introduce the use of pain thermometer/ pain chart.	S.N. King – assisted by Senior Student Mackie	By 30.10.94
Restricted mobility and non-verbal signs of pain displayed.	Set up meeting with physiotherapist to discuss effectiveness and timing of analgesia.	S.N. Ross	By 30.7.94
	Set up a collaborative monitoring exercise which examines patient-centred criteria. O1 & O2 P1 & P2 P6 & P7	S.N. Shepherd Physio Jones	By 31.8.94

important that the action plan is implemented in a structured and systematic manner with, for example, the following provisions included:
- the nature of the changes must be made known to staff
- the date of the introduction of the changes should have been agreed
- the phases of the alteration process ought to be communicated
- colleagues and other professionals should be informed
- the date for subsequent evaluation of the change should be known.

11. Take Action
This step needs no discussion here as it is simply putting into practice the action plan already agreed upon.

12. Re-evaluate the Results
After allowing time for the action plan to be implemented, the audit will be repeated to see whether the action has been effective and if patient care has improved as a result. If the observed action now conforms to the agreed standard, then the action plan has been successfully implemented.

13. Review the Standard
Definitions of quality in the form of standards and criteria need periodic review due to the dynamic nature of quality. The life of any standard is limited and therefore a formal review of the standard needs to take place. At the very least, the following questions need to be asked:
- Is the standard still relevant and useful?
- Does the standard need to be updated?
- Does some new practice, technology, procedure, concept or statutory requirement need to be incorporated into the standard to ensure that it represents up-to-date quality?

Any new ideas or amendments now need to be incorporated into the standard and further implement/achieve by and review dates set. The circle has now been completed and a new standard developed.

Support Structure
This section describes how groups are organised in order to support decentralised standard setting activities. A support structure with clear roles, responsibilities and functions is needed so that this quality improvement activity can be successfully accomplished (Figure 1.4.9).

The system is based at ward or unit level, or in the community, the group may be either a locally based primary health-care team or a geographically based group of, for example, community nurses. The charge nurse/senior nurse should take responsibility for:
- setting up the team
- arranging meetings
- being actively involved in each of the stages of the cycle
- reporting activities to senior managers at other levels of the organisation.

The team consists of representatives from the ward staff including health-care assistants and students. In addition, a nurse teacher and any other interested volunteers, including patients, may participate. Often, as a way of saving time, the structure developed dictates that the standard setting team represents staff from three or four wards, for example surgical wards may develop a standard on pain management together. If this is the case, time still needs to be invested at ward level gaining ideas and feeding back progress to ensure commitment and implementation of the standard.

No more than eight people should be in a team and the members should be volunteers and be prepared to stay in the team for the duration of the whole activity. Meetings should be arranged at staff's convenience, within working hours, at least once a month with the duration of the meeting dependent on local circumstances and the purpose of the meeting. It is important that the meetings are held on a regular basis, to update on progress and ensure effective communication both within the team and with other members of staff. The team leader should plan the meetings well in advance and be strict in relation to starting and finishing times. Staff may prepare work outside meeting times and then discuss it at the meetings.

Initially the team will require the assistance of a facilitator (see below) to ensure that the group becomes established and that progress is made in the right direction. The role of the facilitator is to support local groups through all stages of the quality assurance cycle. The activity of the ward or primary health-care team needs to be co-ordinated in a manner which ensures that information on quality assurance and standards of care is shared throughout the trust or health board/authority.

Effective communication and support can be achieved by ensuring that groups are established at the various levels within the organisation (Figure 1.4.9). The most important interactions take place between the organisational level and the local level with reports on activities being given to the management team. This ensures that any nursing quality assurance initiatives can be developed in the light of other quality objectives and targets at the top of the organisation. An example of how this can work in practice can be found in Part Two, Chapter Three. Due to the time and effort required for quality assurance programmes there is a need to link local activity with the objectives and targets of organisation, but this needs to be handled sensitively so that priorities identified by staff are not compromised.

The standard setting team has seven major tasks:
– select areas for quality improvement
   formulate criteria, agree standard
– measure criteria
– evaluate results
– plan corrective action
– re evaluate activity
– report to quality assurance co-ordinating group.

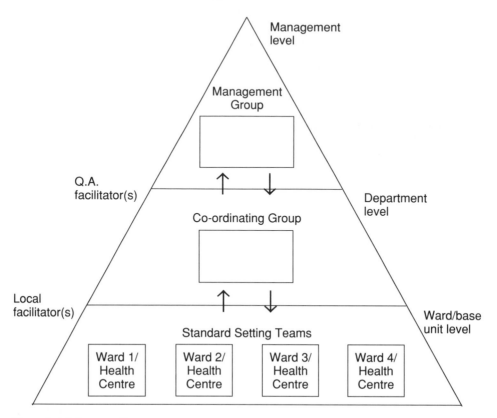

Figure1.4.9 *Support Structure*

Study Activity 7.

Choose a current standard setting activity in one clinical area where you have had experience.

a. How was the subject selected?

b. Was the standard developed to improve quality?

c. Did the activity involve other health care professionals apart from nurses?

The Quality Assurance Co-ordinating Group

This group supports the activities of the standard setting team at local level. The group can be set up to cover geographical or specialty areas (for instance, reviewing quality of orthopaedic care covering four wards within two hospitals or considering a range of surgical specialties within one hospital). Membership of the co-ordinating group includes the nursing director, or person with delegated authority for quality within nursing, representatives from each local team, a representative from education, the facilitator and lay representation.

The co-ordinating group has four functions:
- examine standards and criteria to identify any management support required, including additional resources
- support and co-ordinate activities at local level
- write organisational standards
- report to the management group responsible for quality assurance throughout the organisation.

The Quality Assurance Management Group

Since the establishment of NHS trusts the name and composition of the group at the management or organisational level of the structure can vary from place to place. Its members may include: the quality assurance manager, the chairperson of the clinical audit committee, clinical directors, business managers and lay representatives.

The management group has six main functions:
- receive reports from quality co-ordinating groups
- link quality assurance information with operational and strategic plans, including purchaser quality specifications
- report quality initiatives to trust board and purchasers
- identify areas for quality improvement at organisational and local level
- maintain an effective information system, including the indexing of standards
- maintain an effective educational programme.

The composition and the function of groups carrying out quality assurance activity have been outlined. These can only be taken as a guide and each area will develop its own to reflect its philosophy and purpose. The key elements to consider are as follows:
- groups are identified with clear functions
- a full programme of meetings is arranged in advance
- representation and documentation are such that clear communication takes place.

Indexing Standards

Central to the co-ordination and dissemination of information on nursing quality assurance initiatives is a system for storing and classifying any standards and criteria that have been agreed. An indexing system first developed in 1985 in West Berkshire Health Authority has been developed further in several other health authorities who have adopted the dynamic approach to quality. The indexing system consists of the following items:
- *Topic List*
  The topics are headings identified primarily by nurses, chosen to reflect the philosophy of care that the nursing system is aiming to provide (see Figure 1.4.2). Other groups, for example paramedical and ancillary staff, have been able to use the categories identified in the nursing index.
- *Sub-topic List*
  The sub-topics reflect the sub-categories falling within each of the major topic

headings. Both the topic and sub-topic lists can be extended to accommodate the experience and needs of the nurse practitioners. For indexing purposes it is relatively easy to classify a large number of locally developed standards using the system. Figure 1.4.10 provides excerpts from the Standards of Care Index from a typical health board.

- *Patient Care Groups*

  The care groups are defined by staff writing the local standard. They may be broad groups, for instance "all elderly patients in the community", or they may be very specific, for instance, "low-risk antenatal mothers".

- *Location*

  The specialty, ward or unit where the standard originated is recorded in the index. This is to help other personnel wishing for more information to contact the standard setting team directly.

- *Review Date*

  Each standard setting team is asked to state when they expect to implement their standard and when they are likely to be in a position to audit it. By making the review date specific, managers can discuss the audit procedure with the facilitator and the ward team. This also alerts staff to standards where the review date has been reached but where no report has been received by the co-ordinating group. Having audited clinical practice, a review should then take place of the written standard.

Recent Developments

A recent three-year research study, funded by the Department of Health and carried out as part of the RCN Standards of Care Research and Development Programme, set out to evaluate the impact of DySSSy on nursing actions and patient outcomes. The design of the study was a multi-centre, quasi-experiment matching acute surgical wards to examine pain management. "The study wished to explore whether and to what extent criteria sets derived from an expert group differed from criteria generated by local practitioner groups." (Kitson et al, 1993) The main findings were:

- "Two of the five local groups had criteria convergence scores of more than 55%, demonstrating that the local knowledge on the topic was acceptable."
- "Unless local groups are properly facilitated, they are less likely to generate criteria that converge to a high degree with the expert criteria".
- "The expert group underwent a much more controlled and systematic approach to the task than any of the local groups who were supported by newly trained facilitators".

Other developments include a series of booklets on specific standards of care, a teaching pack and a software package, all produced by the RCN Standards of Care Project. In addition, the Quality Assurance Network (QUAN) has been established to provide support to all health-care professionals involved in quality assurance.

Conclusion

Achieving a quality service depends as much on people as it does on systems

Figure 1.4.10 *Excerpts from Standards of Care Index*

Excerpts from Standards of Care Index

Reference	Topic, Sub-topic and Standard Statement	Review Date
01- 01/101	**Individualised Care** Systematic Approach to Nursing Care "Each patient receives planned individual care based on a systematic approach"	01.02.94
C1/102	**Individualised Care** Eating and Drinking "Each child has an individualised feeding programme, recorded in his nursing profile notes and followed by all members of staff to ensure continuity of approach to feeding problems from meal to meal"	01.06.94
01/103	**Individualised Care** Mobilising – "Positioning" "Each child has his own individualised positioning programme which is illustrated in his nursing profile and recorded on a daily sheet to ensure continuity throughout the day"	01.10.95
01/104	**Individualised Care** Eliminating "All patients who are incontinent of urine will have a toilet programme to meet their needs and regain continence within their capabilities"	01.12.94
02- 02/101	**Safety** Maintaining a Safe Environment in The Recovery Area (following ECT) "Patients in the Recovery Area will receive competent and individualised post-treatment, post-anaesthetic care"	01.10.95
03- 03/101	**Health Education** Prevention of Post-Operative Complications "Nursing staff have an understanding of the social, psychological and health education needs of patients in the prevention of post-operative complications"	01.06.94

and techniques. Christine Townsend (1992) alerts us to the danger that "New systems for standard setting and inspection will be adopted readily while the necessary attitudes, skills and working relationships go largely ignored and undeveloped." She goes on to say, "Nowhere is this more relevant than in the NHS, which is both a very people-intensive organisation and one in which team working is essential."

The experience of one of the authors has been that, in fact, this has been the case within the NHS where an excessive amount of time and effort is being spent on devising strategies, objectives and systems, with little attention being paid to people. Continuous quality improvement should not be brought about by inspection and standard setting but rather by means of empowerment and skills in problem-solving, and in this respect DySSSy, by embracing management of change principles, has often been successful in creating a culture which combines dynamic standard setting, problem-solving and empowerment. In this chapter the Dynamic Standard Setting System and the support structure needed to facilitate its implementation have been described, the *how* of quality assurance activity. In the next chapter the question as to *who* carries out the activities is considered as the roles of the participants are examined.

References

Donabedian A 1966 *Evaluating the quality of medical care.* Millbank Memorial Fund Quarterly 44: 166-206.

Kendall H, Kitson AL 1986 *Rest assured.* Nursing Times Vol. 82 No. 35: 19-21.

Kendall H 1988 *The West Berkshire approach.* Nursing Times Vol. 84 No. 27 33-34.

Kitson A L, Harvey G, Hyndman S, Yerrell P 1993 *A comparison of expert- and practitioner-derived criteria for post-operative pain management.* Journal of Advanced Nursing 18: 218-232.

Lang N M 1976 A Model for Quality Assurance in Nursing *in*: Vansell Davidson S, PSRO utilization and audit in patient care. CV Mosby, St Louis.

McFarlane J 1970 The Proper Study of the Nurse, RCN Standards of Nursing Care. RCN, London.

Øvretveit J 1992 Health Service Quality. Blackwell Scientific Publications, Oxford.

Royal College of Nursing 1989 A Framework for Quality. Scutari, Harrow.

Royal College of Nursing 1980 Standards of Nursing Care. RCN, London.

Royal College of Nursing 1981 Towards Standards. RCN, London.

Royal College of Nursing 1990 Quality Patient Care: An Introduction to RCN Dynamic Standard Setting System (DySSSy). Scutari, London.

Scherer K 1985 *Satisfaction guaranteed.* Nursing Times Vol. 81 No. 22: 32-33.

Schroeder PS and Maibusch RM 1984 Nursing Quality Assurance – A Unit-based Approach. Aspen Systems Corporation, Rockville, MD.

Townsend C 1992 in: Øvretveit J op. cit.

World Health Organization 1982 Development of Standards of Nursing Practice: Report on WHO Meeting, Sonvollen, Norway, 6-9 December, ICP/HSR048.

World Health Organization 1984 Preparation of Guidelines for Standards of Nursing Practice: Report on a WHO Working Group, Brussels, 22-25 October ICP/HSR 302/MOI.

Further Reading

Catterson J 1988 *Quality assurance: a model for nursing*. Senior Nurse Vol. 8 No. 6: 24-25.

Crawford M 1989 *Setting standards in occupational therapy*. British Journal of Occupational Therapy 52(8).

Donabedian A 1989 *Institutional and professional responsibilities in quality assurance*. Quality Assurance in Health Care Vol. 1 No. 1.

Ellis R 1989 Professional Competence and Quality Assurance in the Caring Professions. Chapman and Hall, London.

Five Regional Consortium Ltd 1991 Using Information in Managing the Nursing Resource (Rainbow Pack). Greenhalgh and Co. Ltd.

Howell J and Marr H 1988 *Visible improvements*. Nursing Times Vol. 84 No. 25: 33-34.

Kitson A L 1988 *Raising the standards*. Nursing Times Vol. 84 No. 25: 28-32.

Macdonald M 1991 Scottish Nursing Standards Project Report.

Marr H 1991 Case Study 11, Quality and Life in A Guide to Total Quality Management. Scottish Enterprise, Glasgow.

Marr H 1991 Establishing Standards of Care in Nursing. Scottish Further Education Unit Case Study, Glasgow.

Marr H and Pirie M 1989 *Protecting privacy*. Nursing Times Vol. 86 No. 13: 58-59

Padilla G V and Grant M M 1982 *Quality assurance programme for nursing*. Journal of Advanced Nursing 7: 135-145.

Royal College of Nursing 1987 In Pursuit of Excellence: A Position Statement on Nursing. RCN, London.

Royal College of Nursing 1989 Standards of Care Series. Management in Nursing. Scutari Projects, Harrow.

Stevens P J M, Schade A L, Chalk B, Slevin O D'A 1993 Understanding Research. Campion Press, Edinburgh.

The British Dietetic Association 1993 Setting and Monitoring Standards in the Workplace. Professional Development Committee Briefing Paper No. 7.

5 The Key Players

Introduction

This chapter explores the roles which the key players have in quality assurance activity. Whether experienced or just starting out, client or manager, there is a part for each one to play in the striving for the best possible health care at the lowest possible cost.

One definition of quality previously stated is "meeting the customer's requirements", but who is the customer in the Health Service?
It may be the purchaser of the service (Health Board/Authority, GP fundholder).
It may be the recipient of the service (patient/client).
It may be the internal customer (employee of the service).

Learning Outcomes

After studying this chapter the reader should be able to:
– define who the customer is within health care;
– outline the role of nurses in quality improvement activity;
– describe the role of students of nursing in quality
  improvement activity;
– describe the role of patients and lay people in the three
  phases of the quality assurance cycle;
– list the requirements necessary for the lay person to be
  actively involved in the three phases;
– list the three dimensions of health service quality outlined
  by Øvretveit;
– appreciate the complexity of how clients' perceptions are
  formed;
– describe the role of the manager in centrally and locally
  organised methods of quality assurance activities;
– describe how purchasing can contribute to quality in health
  care;
– describe two skills which nurses may bring to purchasing
  care.

The Role of the Nurse

If quality assurance is about the carrying out of professional work by qualified people then the role and contribution of the nurse is of paramount importance in this activity. As professionals, nurses have to guard against being complacent and protectionist about their practice, otherwise the need and ability to evaluate their own practice and consider other ways of thinking and working may be absent from their more important agendas.

It has been said many times that involvement in the change process is necessary to foster commitment to the change. In the implementation of locally organised activities nurses have a great deal of involvement, although this may not be the case in centrally organised activities (as, for instance, in the application of Phaneuf's Audit). It should be mentioned, however, that the application of Monitor does include asking nurses about the quality of nursing and sometimes the charge nurse may become an assessor. In locally organised activities, the degree of involvement can be greater in all stages of the process, setting the criteria, measuring and taking action.

> **Study Activity 1.**
> Consider how the contribution of the nurse may be maximised in centrally organised activity as, for instance, in the implementation of Monitor. Discuss in your group.

For any quality assurance activity to be successful staff require the necessary skills and knowledge to participate effectively in the process, and therefore training needs to have a high priority. Øvretveit (1990) observes that: "Successful quality programmes pay as much attention to changing human relationships between managers and staff, and staff and patients as to introducing new systems, specification, and measurement. There needs to be as much emphasis on changing people's attitude towards their work as on training them to use specific tools and techniques. Tools are only used if people want to use them. They are only used correctly if people have been trained to use them and have the time to do so."

Of course, once staff are given the tools which help them evaluate their practice, the need for learning and training becomes even greater as they are faced with areas within their practice which they can improve upon. Proponents of quality assurance all agree that creating a learning climate has to be an urgent priority for any organisation. Recent research on skill mix and quality of care reinforces this. "Finally, the results have been related to current debates about staff and skill substitution and the use of support staff. The variations in both quality and outcome with higher grade staff suggest that investment in employing qualified staff, providing post-qualification training and developing effective methods of organising nursing care appeared to pay dividends in the delivery of good-quality patient care." (Carr-Hill, 1992.)

Historically, ongoing learning and updating has often been an area which has been neglected within nursing, and therefore it may be worth while pausing here to identify some of the issues contributing to the question of updating practice and consider how they are being resolved.

Nurses' salaries account for more than half the total budget and nurses are the largest single discipline within the Health Service. Despite this, however, the percentage of manpower time allocated for education and training has traditionally been low. At the point of delivery generally speaking, although changes in knowledge and practice are taking place at an ever-increasing pace, there has been a lack of both peer review and cost-effective mechanisms put in place to keep up to date. For instance, attendance at conferences and study days may not be exploited fully by means of objective setting, applying the achieved learning outcomes to practice and a general sharing with colleagues of any newly acquired information or knowledge.

> **Study Activity 2.**
> Find out how in-service and post-basic training is organised in your clinical area. Is there:
> – a standard or policy?
> – a person responsible?
> – a programme?
> – a budget?
> Discuss in your group.

Nurse training in the past did not encourage questioning and did not regard learning as a lifelong activity in contrast to current educational thinking. The Audit Commission's report, *Making Best Use of Ward Nursing Resources*, highlights the need for additional education and training and concludes that "Good quality nursing care requires not only that the staffing of wards is adequate but also that nurses are equipped with the right skills and education to adapt to modern care requirements." (1991)

Project 2000 A New Preparation for Practice (UKCC 1986) holds the key to facilitating changes in education and attitudes to learning. First introduced in 1989, this new preparation for practice has been phased in throughout the United Kingdom, bringing benefits for patients, and equipping nurses to meet the changing health needs into the 21st century.

The recently updated *Code of Professional Conduct* (UKCC1992) distributed to every registered nurse is more directive in its approach by replacing the word "shall" by "must" – *"You are personally accountable for your practice and, in the exercise of your professional accountability, must: maintain and improve your professional knowledge and competence."*

> **Study Activity 3.**
> Examine your copy of the Code of Professional Conduct. Select only one responsibility and show how this should be accomplished in practical terms.

Furthermore, proposals by the UKCC have introduced *Post Registration Education and Practice* (PREP) (UKCC), which outlines the statutory requirement for post basic education and training within nursing. To maintain their registration and right to practise, nurses must complete a minimum of five days of study leave every three years. Although it is hoped that all nurses can be phased into the scheme by 1996, it is yet unclear who will fund nurses to undertake the required study days.

The single most important element, however, which could underwrite the changes in this vital area is a change in attitude to the value and importance of learning by the individual and the organisation - an attitude which is creative, facilitative and opportunistic. An acknowledgement by top management that education is at the heart of any successful quality programme is the essential requirement which would demonstrate their commitment to quality assurance activities.

The Role of the Student Nurse

Although professional practice may play the key role in quality assurance activity, students of nursing also have their part to play. Their contribution to quality assurance should be incorporated into their learning process so that they gain knowledge and practical experience of quality assurance methods.

One way of making a useful contribution, especially for senior students, can be in the initial identification of desirable standards within the clinical area. Their involvement and participation as part of a standard setting team will certainly lead to a greater commitment to the standard, particularly with regard to their special contribution - new-found knowledge. This recently acquired knowledge offered by student nurses has often contributed to the updating of practising nurses within a clinical setting and, although this is not desirable, it has often been relied upon in the past.

In a similar fashion, students can make a valuable contribution during the auditing and taking action phases in locally organised quality assurance activity. The student nurse's introduction to learning about quality assurance activity should be dealt with at an early stage in the curriculum. Colleges of nursing and health studies will also have their own quality assurance programmes, to maintain and improve standards of education and the learning environment. Students will therefore have many opportunities to learn about quality assurance activity as they play their part as consumers of the service.

> **Study Activity 4.**
> **a.** As a student nurse discuss in your group any contribution you may have made to standard setting/quality improvement activity in the clinical area.
> **b.** Discuss any contribution you have made to quality assurance within the college, for example completion of questionnaire, post-course interview.

The Role of the Patient

In the previous two sections we have considered the roles of nurses and of nursing students in quality assurance activities. Important as these roles are, it must be remembered that patients themselves have the central part to play as consumers of the service. Their feedback and involvement in defining and redefining quality is essential in order to develop a service which is tailored to *meet the customers' requirements.* They are the end customers and the judgement of quality received is entirely in their hands.

Donabedian (1980) has defined quality as the goodness of technical care, the goodness of the interpersonal relationship and the goodness of the amenities. (see also Figure 1.1.3). Although patients cannot be expected to judge the technical aspects of care in an informed way, they have every right to comment on the quality of the interpersonal relationship and the amenities as they have experienced them. Traditionally, it has been the role of the professionals to agree on the standard of care to be achieved as, apart from other considerations, patients are not always in the position of knowing what they need and therefore quality cannot be defined only in terms of customer satisfaction and expressed consumer demand. Øvretveit (1990) points out that consumer or client quality is only one important dimension of service quality and suggests that it is the integration of client quality, professional quality and management quality that is necessary in order to arrive at a satisfactory definition. He stresses the importance of the patient's role when he states that service quality is about client perceptions - "Health providers now need to understand more about how clients perceive health services in general and their service in particular, and make changes to respond to these perceptions" (op. cit.) Furthermore, he suggests "that a client's perceptions of a health service are formed in even more complex ways and are made up of the following:

– what clients *want* from the service, that is, what they would like to receive from it, and what they feel it *should* ideally provide. (We note that clients rarely ask for this from the service by making a *demand.*)
– what clients *expect* the service will provide, that is, what they think it *would* provide
– what clients think they *need*, which may be different from what they want ("I know it's good for me, but what I really want is...")
– their perceived *experience* of the service at different times
– their global and *enduring perception* of the service, the perceived quality" (op. cit.)

One intention of the Health Service reforms was to widen choice and make services more responsive to clients. This of course may still be interpreted by a practitioner from a professional perspective with the service being responsive to need as identified by the professional, traditionally the one who knows best.

It has been advocated for some time now that quality groups at all levels within health-care organisations should include lay people, and this is now becoming a reality. Gradually, and not before time, involvement of the patient and members of the general public is increasing significantly and mechanisms are now in place locally to systematically gather information and to take account of feedback and public opinion. Involvement of health councils, user groups and liaison committees are facilitating this process. In addition, these groups are becoming increasingly involved with the developing of purchaser quality specifications.

The Patient's Charter calls for continuing efforts to improve standards of health care and advocates that everyone, *including users and consumers of the service*, has to be involved in the process of setting standards. Having outlined the role of the patient in the describing phase of the quality assurance cycle, we can now turn to the auditing and taking action phases.

Consumers have participated in the auditing or measuring phase for some considerable time now, knowingly or unknowingly, principally by involvement in consumer surveys as respondents. Following an episode of care, cards for suggestions or complaints are provided to give valuable feedback for both practitioners and management. However, it is time that consumers came to the other side of the clipboard and participated in the observation and questioning alongside the professionals rather than simply being the sources or suppliers of the data.

> **Study Activity 5.**
> Find out how feedback about the service is gathered in your clinical area. Look for examples of:
> questionnaires;
> post-care interviews;
> mechanisms for suggestions/complaints;
> thank-you/appreciation cards.

In the past the taking action phase has certainly not involved clients, and it may need a major shift in attitude by both professionals and consumers for it to take place. Lay people can become involved in initiating the change, the action planning, decision-making and reviewing that the action plan has, in fact, been successfully implemented. In order for this to be meaningful the following requirements are needed:
- having an opinion and being willing to voice it
- being constructively critical
- being empowered.

In conclusion, there is now a realisation with the implementation of quality strategies and programmes that the most important item being demanded to shape the service is customer feedback. In many arenas the attitude that no news is good news has gone, but we still have a long way to go. Words and actions are inconsistent and, even where such values are being expounded, feedback, and particularly complaints, are still feared, brushed under the carpet and rationalised. We need to reach the stage when they are welcomed and treated as a necessity.

Study Activity 6.

Discuss in your group how complaints procedures are handled in your clinical area:
- is there a written procedure?
- does the procedure identify who, how and time-scales for dealing with complaints?

The following was a comment made by an "enlightened" practice nurse at a recent workshop. Another member of the workshop group was describing a visit to her GP's surgery and remarked on the gatekeeping behaviour of the receptionist, suggesting that what the receptionist needed was more appropriate training to encourage a more receptive attitude. The "enlightened" practice nurse defended the attitude and behaviour of the receptionist and explained how she understood the difficulties that the receptionist faced, as she herself worked in a surgery. Her solution was to suggest that patients ought to have the opportunity to spend the day behind the receptionist's desk in order to gain understanding of the receptionist's work and to appreciate the difficulties she faced. One of the authors is rather saddened that she had missed the point of "a client-centred service", and thought it would be a better exercise for the receptionist to spend a day in the waiting room of the surgery!

Study Activity 7.

Shadowing someone at work for a short time often provides the opportunity for greater appreciation and understanding of her role. Have you had the opportunity or can you be given the opportunity to shadow someone within the clinical area? Discuss in the group what you learned or would want to learn from the experience.

The Role of the Manager

It is the manager in quality assurance activity who is charged with creating the organisational framework within which the activity can take place. It is important that management supports quality assurance by making it an integrated part of everyday practice, whether it be centrally or locally organised. This involves providing resources, such as time to carry out quality improvement programmes organising secretarial and any other ancillary backup which may be needed, and in general creating a climate which encourages and supports such initiatives (Marr, 1992).

The manager's role in centrally organised activity is usually to carry out and co-ordinate methods or have an accountable member of staff who is responsible for quality assurance. This includes selection of a suitable tool, setting up a training programme and often being an assessor during the auditing phase. The manager also has a key role to play in the preparation of staff before centrally organised activity is undertaken. In addition, the manager must ensure that there is an effective system in place to feed back the findings of the exercise to the team members. In the taking action phase there needs to be a commitment to desirable, but at the same time, realistic goals for implementation. Where strengths and areas of good practice have been identified the manager is in a strong position both to give recognition to the staff and to set up effective communication to share such practices in a non-threatening way.

Study Activity 8.

a. Discuss in your group how quality assurance is organised and who is responsible for its implementation in your clinical area.

b. Discuss in your group how quality assurance is organised and who is responsible for its implementation where you are studying.

In locally organised activity, the manager's duties have been defined in the following way though the list is not exhaustive. It should be noted here that the comments which follow this list of duties have resulted from the experiences of one of the authors, and the list and the remarks are not intended to be complete or prescriptive. They are included as a practical *ad hoc* guide for those involved in quality assurance programmes.

– *Support and encourage staff within one's sphere of responsibility*
It is interesting to note how often staff look to their manager for a sign that this is a worthwhile activity. Positive encouragement and guidance from a manager can counteract lack of interest and help nursing staff find time for activities. If something is perceived as being worthwhile then time can be found even in the busiest of places. Managers can assist here both in the valuing of the activities and in the setting up and maintaining of the support structure. At a recent audit workshop a practising nurse announced that one year before she had been promised a half-day monthly for quality assurance activities by her manager but this had never materialised. Perhaps the question that should be asked here is, was she not given it, or did she not take it? Even one hour per month regularly would be enough to indicate commitment and keep the process moving forward.

Study Activity 9.

Discuss how time and resources are allocated to quality improvement activity in your clinical area.

Include setting standards/quality initiatives in existing unit meeting agendas
This is an ideal way to gently introduce the topic of quality, raise awareness generally and demonstrate that this is "not going to go away". It is also a good opportunity to give air time to those ward/department managers and nurses who are involved in activities to explain what they are doing. This often whets the appetite and promotes healthy competition among those not yet involved. A final advantage of this aspect of management is that it is a good use of time.

It is building on existing activities rather than prematurely setting up a quality meeting probably doomed to failure due to lack of activity and commitment. It is better to have a meeting where the agenda is full rather than a meeting where there is little to report.

– *Communicate with facilitators about quality assurance activities within one's unit and sphere of responsibility*
It is essential for a manager to have a good understanding of the standard setting initiatives that are taking place within her unit and therefore formal communication with local facilitators is essential.This has benefits both for the manager, in that it keeps her informed, and also for the facilitator in the form of support. Local facilitators as practising nurses often find it difficult to free themselves to assist groups in standard setting. This is further compounded if both the group and the facilitator are inexperienced.

– *Participate in standard setting activities by offering expertise, in-service training and preparation in the quality initiative*
The value of education, training and learning has already been highlighted. It is interesting to note the different responses from organisations to this important issue of preparation as it varies from structured workshops and study days for all staff to a "get on and do it" approach. The latter approach is of course unacceptable. Experience has shown that even half a day can be well spent in increasing motivation and gaining understanding in the why, how and what of locally based quality assurance.

– *Facilitate standard setting activities by ensuring that the standard is signed/ ratified by management as soon as possible*
When the initiative was first introduced it was not unknown for written standards to be sent to managers for ratification and for these standards to be gone for anything between one week and eighteen months.They seemed to disappear – a Bermuda Triangle phenomenon. Thinking positively, one can only assume that such managers were hoping to find more expertise and information before they signed on the dotted line or checked the achievability and legitimacy of such a standard. From a more negative viewpoint, fear of the unknown, power shifting and loss of purpose due to the changing role of the practitioner may have also been the reason for not endorsing the written standard. It should be noted, however, that the initial focus of training was on preparing the practitioners rather than nurse managers, with the effect that the latter group was often less informed and less involved.

> **Study Activity 10.**
> Find out the process for ratifying standards in the clinical area.

– *Participate in the identification of areas for quality improvement*
The manager, along with ward or department staff, can identify areas of concern from experience, observation, patient complaints or results of an

audit. Practising nurses almost exclusively select specific areas of concern as the basis for developing standards. It tends to be an outsider - manager, educator, or facilitator - who has an overall and more objective view of the whole situation and who may in fact encourage staff to write a standard about an area of *good* practice.

– *Develop management standards*
  Since practitioners were the initial focus for training in standard setting, the production of management standards has been slow but has gained momentum more recently. Examples of preparatory work in this area are described in the form of a case study in Part Two Chapter Six of this text.

In both centrally and locally organised methods it is important that management shows an interest in the results of the monitoring. This can be done by taking the results seriously and implementing them as widely as possible throughout the organisation. This will stimulate further quality assurance initiatives and motivate staff to pay serious attention to their responsibilities in this area. In this way, it will have a positive impact on the continuation of the process. Experience has shown that when quality assurance activity does not evoke any response from management, motivation becomes stagnant and negative, and eventually quality assurance may be seen as a waste of time. This can also happen when management becomes overinvolved with the content of the initiative and begins making unreasonable demands. Quality assurance might then be seen in a very negative light. This phenomenon is described in detail in the American literature on quality assurance in nursing (Lang, 1976, Schroeder, 1991, Phaneuf, 1976). Despite these difficulties, as long as management maintains a stimulating, interested and committed attitude, quality assurance can become a cost-effective instrument for improving nursing practice.

The Role of the Facilitator

Having explored a number of roles within successful standard setting it would be remiss to leave this topic without at least outlining the role of the facilitator, as it would appear that this often informal role has had a major contribution to make towards the success or failure of standard setting and quality improvement within health care. The facilitator is one who enables individuals working in groups to achieve their goals, by improving group processes and by developing team dynamics. The facilitator's prime concern is not the content of the standard itself; rather it is to enable the group to develop the standard themselves, and in order to achieve this the facilitator avoids active involvement in the content of the team's efforts.

Burnard (1989) has identified the following personal qualities which are needed for interpersonal effectiveness: warmth, genuineness, empathetic understanding, unconditional positive regard and interpersonal skills. Further work on the dimensions of facilitation styles has been developed extensively by Heron (1989).

In DySSSy's early development, three levels of facilitators were perceived as necessary to establish and maintain the Dynamic Standard Setting System in nursing, as in the following extract from the RCN Standards of Care document (Kitson, 1988):

a. Expert facilitator in quality assurance methods
b. Key facilitator within district/hospital health-care setting
c. Local facilitator(s) in a particular specialty within a health-care setting.

The Role of the Expert Facilitator

The expert facilitator is often found working in a national organisation with responsibility for setting up a programme of activity.

Seven key functions have been identified:

1. Introduce the concept of quality assurance to groups of nurses and other health-care workers at every level of the organisation and in every specialty.
2. Develop teaching material for groups wishing to start setting and monitoring quality.
3. Act as consultant to nurses who wish to use the dynamic approach.
4. Be available for ongoing consultation.
5. Run courses to train key facilitators.
6. Develop a system to co-ordinate nursing quality assurance activities on a national level.
7. Develop and train key facilitators.

The Role of the Key Facilitator

The key facilitator operates within a district health authority setting or in a large hospital/primary care complex. Her role is to act as the "internal facilitator" following the initial contact with the expert facilitator who is always seen in an "external" role. Nurses who become key facilitators often come from a research or education background and may be working in a support post, on a special project or in quality assurance. One common denominator is that they are all committed to improving nursing practice. They may start off facilitating one group and quickly become interested in spreading the idea to colleagues. If a key facilitator is identified early on in an organisation the expert facilitator is able to hand over the detailed development planning work to her.

Six main functions have been identified:

1. Teaching
 – provide general information to students on basic nursing courses, in-service training on quality assurance and standards
 – respond to specific requests from staff to start writing standards.
 – support, guide, direct practitioners identified as local facilitators.
 – organise in-depth training days for local facilitators.

2. Setting up the System
 – respond to requests for help from clinical staff who wish to set standards and monitor care
 – act as a facilitator to new groups

- keep managers informed of developments
- explain overall structure, roles and responsibilities of various staff members
- organise first meeting at each organisational level
- offer feedback to staff and guidance on performance.

3. Keeping the System Going
- solve problems - *organisational*, e.g. what is "local level"; interpersonal, e.g. how to stop people from using the system for their own ends; *political*, e.g. how to guard against people sabotaging the system.

4. Integrating Standards and Quality with Other Systems
- quality as management objectives - distinct yet part of management
- relationship between quality and policy and procedure committees
- use regular meetings, e.g. ward sister/nurse manager meetings to include "quality" on the agenda
- reduce conflict or use it constructively between "top-down" and "bottom-up" systems.

5. Giving Feedback
- recognise the importance of demonstrating improvements and effects of change
- set up a standards of care index
- ensure communication systems are working effectively.

6. Keeping One Step Ahead
- central role of key facilitator is to introduce new ideas to local facilitators
- identify topic areas requiring thorough investigation and rigorous methodology.

The Role of the Local Facilitator
Depending upon the size and complexity of the health-care organisation, the local facilitator role may be highly developed or there may be more reliance on the key facilitator to support developments. Local facilitators are committed practitioners with an interest in improving the quality of the care they deliver, and who are prepared to work with one or two standard groups within their specialty to help set up the quality assurance system. They must be recognised as expert practitioners in their own specialism, credible practitioners and good communicators.

Local facilitators have at least four key functions :
1. Liaise with key facilitator.
2. Attend unit/ward meetings and facilitate practitioners in setting and monitoring standards.
3. Provide guidance and advice to practitioners both in content of criteria and standards and in format of information.
4. Help sustain interest at local level by putting on lunch-time sessions, study afternoons, working with key facilitator.

The local facilitator may find herself devoting between a half-day and one day per week to this work whilst the key facilitator, depending on the number of groups to develop, may find herself devoting almost all her working time to facilitation and evaluation work. There must be a mechanism within the organisation to permit this kind of development to happen and it is the role of the manager to ensure this takes place.

As DySSSy has developed interprofessionally and is now integrated with other quality systems, the key facilitator is often the Director of Quality and Patient Services or someone accountable to her. Although most likely to have a nursing background, this person will be responsible for quality throughout the organisation.

The Purchaser–Provider Relationship

One of the most significant government reforms in *Working for Patients* (op. cit.) has been the development of the purchaser–provider relationship within a contractual setting. The purchasers of health care are the health boards, health authorities and GP fundholders; the providers of health care are the hospital trusts and directly managed units.

At a recent health-care conference Virginia Bottomley underlined the importance of the role of purchasers: "From first to last, it is the purchasers who should be in control. They pay the piper, they must call the tune." (1993) In general, the overall guiding principle of purchasers is that resources should be used with the sole purpose of improving health services for patients and the health of the public as a whole.

Health-care services should be purchased only from organisations which set and maintain high standards of care and service. These organisations should also demonstrate a total approach to quality assurance which is systematic but which also provides opportunities for innovation.

In particular, purchasers of care have responsibility for:
– assessing the health needs of their local population
– specifying the service required; the specification must take account of cost, volume, activity and quality
– agreeing a contract with a provider who will deliver the specified service
– monitoring and reviewing the contract.

Benton and Smith (1992) believe that "monitoring quality specifications is an essential role of the purchasing team" and encourage "more individuals to grasp the opportunity to develop and fulfil this much needed role".

A recent study (King's Fund, 1992) set out to identify the nurse's contribution to purchasing. The skills which were found to be necessary include:
– the ability to speak in a "range of languages", i.e. the skill to communicate effectively with doctors, lay people and managers, thus bridging the gap between the various groups involved in purchasing and providing care;
– the ability to "understand the business", i.e. "the way different services within and beyond the Health Service can and should mesh together" (ibid.).

"Nurses' strength lies very much in their ability to envisage change and this could be an enormous asset in purchasing, much of which in future will consist of persuading providers to do things differently" (ibid.).

Conclusion

This chapter has considered the contribution of the participants in quality assurance activities at both local and central levels. It is interesting to note that knowledge, skills and attitudes developed while implementing DySSSy are proving to be invaluable in the contribution of quality to the purchasing process, thus facilitating effective collaboration in a trusting relationship to achieve the best possible service at the lowest possible cost.

> **Study Activity 11.**
>
> Identify one aspect of care in the clinical area which is being addressed as a quality improvement initiative and is also specified as a standard within the purchaser quality specifications .
> - Find out how this aspect of care is being monitored and by whom.

References

Audit Commission 1991 The Virtue of Patients: Making Best Use of Ward Nursing Resources. National Health Service, London.

Benton D and Smith M 1992 *Quality monitoring: its role in purchasing.* Nursing Standard Vol. 6 No. 41.

Bottomley V in Mawhinney B 1993 Purchasing for Health. A Framework for Action. NHS Management Executive, London.

Burnard P 1989 Teaching Interpersonal Skills: A Handbook of Experiential Learning for Health Professionals. Chapman & Hall, London.

Carr-Hill R, Dixon R, Gibbs I et al 1992 Skill Mix and the Effectiveness of Nursing Care. University of York, York.

Donabedian A 1980 Explorations in Quality Assessment and Monitoring. Volume 1: The Definition of Quality and Approaches to its Assessment. Health Administration Press, Ann Arbor, Michigan.

Heron J 1989 The Facilitator's Handbook. Kogan Page, London.

King's Fund College 1992 The Professional Nursing Contribution to Purchasing. NHSME, London.

Kitson A L 1988 Role of the Facilitator in Quality Assurance/DySSSy. RCN Standards of Care, London.

Lang N M 1976 A Model for Quality Assurance in Nursing in: Van Sell Davidson S–PSRO utilization and audit in patient care. C V. Mosby, St Louis.

Marr H 1992 *Motivating staff to higher standards.* Nursing Standard Vol. 7 No. 11· 31-34.

NHS in Scotland 1991 The Patient's Charter. A Charter for Health. The Scottish Office, Edinburgh.

Øvretvelt J 1990 Quality Health Services. Brunel University of West London.

Phaneuf M C 1976 The Nursing Audit – Self regulation in nursing practice. Appleton-Century-Crofts, New York.

Schroeder P 1991 *in*: The Encyclopedia of Nursing Care Quality. Aspen Publishers, Gaithersburg, MD.
UKCC 1992 Code of Professional Conduct. UKCC, London.
UKCC 1986 Project 2000: A New Preparation for Practice. UKCC, London.

Further Reading

Collard R 1989 Total Quality. Success Through People.Institute of Personnel Management, London.
DOH 1993 A Vision for the Future. NHS Management Executive.
DOH 1993 The Quality Journey. NHS Management Executive.
Drennan D 1992 Transforming Company Culture. McGraw-Hill Book Co., New York.
Groenman N H, Slevin O D'A, Buckenham M 1992 Social and Behavioural Sciences for Nurses. Campion Press, Edinburgh.
Lovelock H 1992 Managing Services. Marketing, Operations and Human Resources, 2nd ed. Prentice-Hall, Englewood Cliffs, NJ.
Normann R 1991 Service Management. 2nd ed. John Wiley & Sons, Chichester.

PART TWO

1　A Nursing Audit Calendar

This case study provides an overview of one facilitator's audit calendar developed from local standards (Figure 2.1.1). It covers one year's activity and was implemented throughout the hospitals where she is Nurse Practice Adviser. Two extracts from the calendar are described below. The first one is concerned with the named nurse initiative and the second with maintaining skin integrity.

Figure 2.1.1 *Nursing Audit Calendar – 1993*

Month	Standard	Persons Responsible
January	Care Planning	1 representative per ward
February		
March	Pressure Area Care	1 representative per ward
April	Named Nurse	1 representative per ward
May	Discharge Planning	1 representative per ward
June		
July	Administration of IV Drugs	1 representative per ward
August		
September	One Nurse Drug Administration	1 representative per ward
October		
November	Care Planning	1 representative per ward
December		

The Named Nurse Audit

As previously described in Part One Chapter Two, the allocation of one responsible nurse for the assessment, planning and evaluation of each individual patient's care has become an important focus of activity in the nursing profession. The basis for the audit described below can be found in *The New Patient's Charter Standard* 8, *viz.*

"A named nurse, midwife or health visitor will be responsible for your nursing or midwifery care."

The case study outlines the background provided to staff, the audit activity, findings and recommendations made.

What needs to be acknowledged is that the named nurse approach is not new; in fact it has been advocated by the Royal College of Nursing for many years. Primary nursing and team nursing have also promoted the importance of patients having a named nurse.

The value of the named nurse being included within *The Patient's Charter* is that it shows that the Government has recognised the contribution of having an individual qualified nurse caring for a patient. The Audit Commission (1991) emphasised the importance of continuity of care, and this has been supported by numerous research studies that demonstrate the value of skilled nursing care in minimising surgical mortality and morbidity, reducing length of stay and preventing re-admission (Buchan et al, 1991; RCN,1992; Bagust, 1992).

Within these particular hospitals, implementation of this standard was not a difficult task, due to the commitment and enthusiasm of its nurses. All wards were already practising team nursing so patients were aware of who was caring for them, and primary nursing was due to be piloted in 1993 on one of the wards.

Team nursing ensures that, on admission, every patient is allocated a named qualified nurse. This nurse becomes the patient's named nurse, and plans care with the patient, the family or significant other. This care is documented in a care plan which is kept at the patient's bedside. The named nurse ensures that her name is recorded on the nursing care plan. Some wards encourage the patient to sign his care plan so that he becomes an active partner in his nursing care.

When the named nurse goes off duty, she hands over to the deputy named nurse in the presence of the patient. This ensures that the patient's care needs are communicated clearly and that the patient knows who will be looking after him.

The standard on the named nurse was written by a small group of nurses and then sent to all areas for comment. Once the final draft was agreed, a baseline audit took place in October 1992 (Figure 2.1.2).

Figure 2.1.2 *Audit Form for Named Nurse*

Audit Objective   To find out if patients are aware of the nurse caring for them.
Sample   20% random sample per ward area
Time Frame   1 day
Auditor(s)   Nurse Practice Adviser

TARGET GROUP	METHOD	CODE	AUDIT CRITERIA
Nurses	Ask	S1b	Are posts filled to establishment?
Nurses	Observe	S2 & O2	Is the nurse wearing a name badge?
		S3	Is a system of team/primary nursing in progress?
		P1	Does the patient have a care plan?
Records	Observe	P3	Did the named nurse undertake the initial assessment?
		P4	Does the care plan show who the named nurse is?
		O3a	Is the assessment written by the named nurse?
		O3b	Is the assessment signed by the named nurse?
Patient	Ask	P1 & O1	Are you aware of your named nurse?
		P2 & P5	Did the nurse introduce him/herself to you?

The audit results are given in Figure 2.1.3

Figure 2.1.3 *Audit Results*

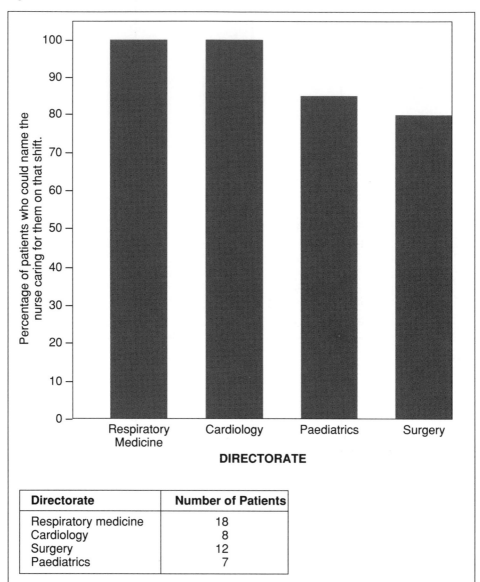

Directorate	Number of Patients
Respiratory medicine	18
Cardiology	8
Surgery	12
Paediatrics	7

* The two surgical patients who were unaware of their named nurse were being cared for by an agency nurse.

The recommendations which resulted from the audit were as follows:
1. Lead nurses should delegate responsibility to a permanent member of the nursing staff, to ensure that agency nurses are made aware of the named nurse standard.
2. Re-audit standard in May 1993.

Pressure Area Care Audit

In October 1991, a standard setting group was formed because nurses and occupational therapists were concerned about the inadequate provision of pressure-relieving devices to deal with those they had identified as high-risk patients. The purpose of the group was to assist all those involved in the care of patients to reduce the incidence of pressure sores, and to prevent pressure sores from occurring.

Although pressure sores are often regarded as a failure of nursing care, it is now widely recognised that they are an interdisciplinary problem, and pressure sores do not only occur in long-term patients. It is often not realised that the acutely ill patients who suddenly become immobilised are often more at risk of developing sores than the long-term immobile, and this has obvious cost implications for the health authority.

A Grade 4 pressure sore costs approximately £25,000 to treat (Waterlow, 1991). Overall, the annual cost of treating pressure sores is known to be up to £1.5 million per health authority, and it is increasing at a rate of 13% per annum. Another £100,000 to £1,000,000 could be added to this should the authority be sued as a result of patients developing pressure sores during their hospital stay. Pressure sores cause patients a great deal of discomfort and distress. 95% of all pressure sores are preventable (Hibbs, 1988).

Investigation by the standard setting group has shown that many risk factors are involved. The most important of these are the lack of available resources (particularly aids and equipment), lack of knowledge, and the fact that approximately 50% of the patient population falls into an "at risk" group. There was no baseline incidence measurement available so the extent of the problem was unknown.

Over the past six months, a standard (Figure 2.1.4) and an audit form (Figure 2.1.5) have been written and partially implemented. The audit took place on 8th June 1992. The aim was to use the information collected as a baseline for further development.

The report that follows describes the methods used to undertake the audit, the results of the audit, the conclusions drawn from the results and recommendations for action.

Audit Methodology

The following was the information gathered, summarised in an audit form (Figure 2.1.5).

Operational Definitions:

The Waterlow assessment policy is designed as an aid to both prevention and treatment of pressure sores. Scores are allocated to give the patients' risk status.

Figure 2.1.4 *Standard for Pressure Area Care*

Topic	Individual Patient Care	**Implement Standard by**
Sub-Topic	Pressure Area Care	**Audit Standard by**
Care Group	Adult Patients	**Signature of QA Group**
Contact Person		**Signature of Senior Nurse**
		Date
Standard Statement	Nurses identify individual patients at risk from pressure damage and plan care to meet this need to prevent pressure damage from occurring.	

STRUCTURE	PROCESS	OUTCOME
S1. Nurses have the necessary knowledge and skills to use the Waterlow assessment score, and be aware of the causes and prevention of pressure damage.	P1. Patients are allocated to a named nurse on admission to the ward/department.	01. The patient is assessed within one hour of admission to ward/department with evidence in the assessment documentation.
S2. The following resources are available: a) resource file with current research articles b) pressure area care policy. c) Waterlow assessment cards. d) mattress turning and replacement policy.	P2. Every patient is assessed within one hour of admission by the named nurse using the Waterlow assessment tool. Visual inspection of the patient's skin if in an at risk group.	02. The patient's Waterlow score is shown in the care plan.
S3a. Nurses attend lifting technique sessions on induction. S3b. Nurses attend wound care/pressure area care study days within 1 year of employment.	P3. The assessing nurse writes a care plan and commences implementation, following the Waterlow plan. The patient and family are involved in this process.	03. The at risk patient has an up-to-date care plan.
S4. The following pressure area equipment – Spencos, Tendercare, Pegasus, 1 Nimbus bed and Roho cushions are available and functioning.	P4. The interprofessional team is utilised to help with diet, positioning and recreation.	04. The patient can explain his plan of care unless he is medically unable to do this.

Figure 2.1.4 contd. *Standard for Pressure Area Care*

Topic	Individual Patient Care	**Implement Standard by**
Sub-Topic	Pressure Area Care	**Audit Standard by**
Care Group	Adult Patients	**Signature of QA Group**
Contact Person		**Signature of Senior Nurse**
		Date
Standard Statement	Nurses identify individual patients at risk from pressure damage and plan care to meet this need to prevent pressure damage from occurring.	

STRUCTURE	PROCESS	OUTCOME
S5. A record is kept on the ward of any patients with pressure sores so that incidence levels can be monitored.	P5. Pressure relieving devices are used following the assessment, and written in care plan as nursing actions.	05. The incidence of pressure damage is reduced.
S6. A record is kept of patients at risk.	P6. Nurses lift and reposition patients, avoiding shearing and injury.	06. The patient is nursed in bed, or on a chair appropriate (Waterlow plan) to his risk score.
S7. There is a maintenance programme for all equipment/beds on the wards.	P.7 Care is evaluated continuously and particularly when there is a change in the patient's condition, eg. post operatively, haemodynamic instability, administration of narcotic analgesia, prolonged period of fasting.	

Figure 2.1.5 *Audit Form for Pressure Area Care*

Audit Objective	To find out if nurses identify patients at risk of pressure damage and plan their care to prevent this from occurring.		
Sample	44 nurses. 4 nurses per clinical area / 4 patient records / 147 patients		
Time Frame	1 day		
Auditor(s)	Nurse Practice Adviser plus one nurse from each clinical area		
TARGET GROUP	**METHOD**	**CODE**	**AUDIT CRITERIA**
Ward Environment	Observe	S2a S2b S2c	Is there a resource file? Are Waterlow assessment charts available? Is there a mattress turning policy?
Nurses	Ask	S1a S1b S1c	Is the nurse aware of what the Waterlow assessment score is? Can the nurse explain how to use it? Is the nurse aware of the causes of pressure damage?
Records	Observe	P2a & O1 P3a & O2 P3b & P5/O3 P4a P4b	Has the patient been assessed within one hour of admission to the ward? If the patient has been identified as being at risk, has it been identified as a problem? Is there a care plan written following the Waterlow plan? Is there any evidence of family involvement? Has the interprofessional team been involved? If yes, for what reason?
Patient	Ask Observe	O4 O6	Can the patient explain his care plan related to pressure area care? Is the patient being nursed on a bed/chair appropriate to his risk score?

The scores range from:

1-9   = not at risk of developing pressure sores (NAR)
10-14 = at risk of developing pressure sores (AR)
15-19 = high risk of developing pressure sores (HR)
20+   = very high risk of developing pressure sores (VHR)

Depending on the score, the Waterlow policy makes recommendations for nursing care required and prevention aids to be used.

If the patient has a pressure sore, the Waterlow policy provides a staged system from 1-5, as follows:

Blanching hyperaemia	Stage 1	red wound
Non-blanching hyperaemia	Stage 2	red wound, clean but not healed
Ulceration progresses	Stage 3	yellow/infected/inflamed wound
Ulceration extends	Stage 4	infected
Infective necrosis	Stage 5	black/necrotic wound

Audit Results

1. Interviews with nurses.
Sample: 44 nurses of varying grades.
In a convenience sample of 4 nurses per clinical area the following questions were asked:
S1a. Is the nurse aware of what the Waterlow assessment score is?
S1b. Can the nurse explain how to use it?
S1c. Is the nurse aware of the causes of pressure damage?
All nurses met the above criteria.

2. Observed ward environment.
S2a. Is there a resource file?
S2b. Are Waterlow assessment charts available?
S2c. Is there a mattress-turning policy?
All resources identified were in place.
O6. Is the patient being nursed on a bed or chair appropriate to his risk score?
58% of patients were being nursed with the appropriate equipment.

3. Observation of nursing records.
Four sets of nursing records per clinical area were examined.
P3a & O2. If a patient has been identified as being at risk, has it been recognised as a problem?
64% of the patients at risk had this problem identified within the care plan.
P3b, P5 & O3. Is there a care plan written following the Waterlow plan? Is there any evidence of family involvement?
53% of the patients identified at risk had a care plan written following the Waterlow plan.
P4a. Has the interprofessional team been involved?
61% had interprofessional involvement.

4. Assessment and examination of the patients.
The total sample of 147 patients was assessed using the Waterlow assessment policy. If patients had a Waterlow score more than 10, they were physically examined, the presence of pressure sores was staged and the sites recorded.

The Sample (Figure 2.1.6) :
147 in-patients:
17 aged between 0 and 16
130 aged between 17 and 88
Mean age 47
95 male
52 female

73 patients (50% of the population) fell into an at-risk group (Waterlow score more than 10).
Of those, 36 patients (24%) were at high risk and above (Waterlow score greater than 15).
Of the total population, 28 patients, (19%) had pressure sores of which:
13.6% = Stage 1
2.7% = Stage 2
2.7% = Stage 3.
All the patients with pressure sores were identified as at risk.

Figure 2.1.6 *Pressure Area Care Audit Results*

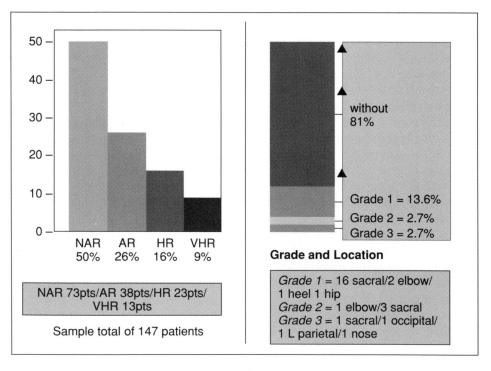

5. Interviews with patients.
In a convenience sample of four patients per clinical area the following question was asked:
O4. Can the patient explain his care plan related to pressure area care?
60% of patients at risk were able to explain their care plan.

6. Inspection of equipment.
A total of 237 mattresses were examined against the following criteria:
   Is the mattress split?
   Is the cover clean?
   Is the foam moist?
   Is the cover wrinkled?
   Does the mattress bottom out?
26 mattresses (11%) were condemnable.
48 mattresses (20%) required review within 3 months.

The audit results illustrate that Grade 1 sacral pressure areas are of concern. Other projects currently in progress may be having a direct impact on this area. For example, lifting and back injuries are currently being explored through a standard setting group because baseline data collected highlighted the lack of lifting aids available on the wards, which could be discouraging nurses from lifting patients.

Figure 2.1.7 *Pilot Study – 10 Patients Receiving Analgesia via a PCA Device*

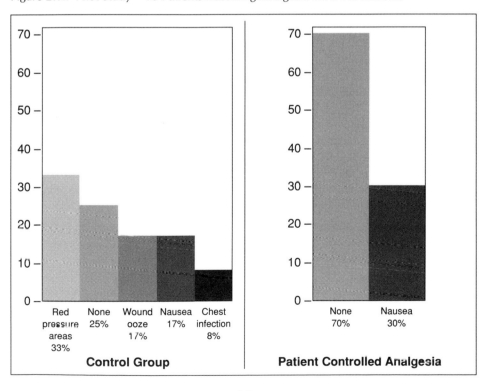

Pain control has also been identified in relation to the development of pressure sores. A pilot study of 10 patients receiving analgesia via a PCA (Patient Controlled Analgesia) device showed that none of them developed pressure sores. The control group developed four (Figure 2.1.7).

Conclusion.

This audit took place to establish a baseline for future audits and to highlight the need to resource complete implementation of the standard. As the audits continue, it will enable correlations to be made between particular groups of patients at risk and the development of pressure sores. This audit has clearly identified problem areas with 50% of the patients on 8th June falling into an *at risk* group and 24% of these patients requiring high-risk equipment such as alternating pressure mattresses and bed systems. Currently the only high-risk equipment available is in the intensive therapy unit, yet clearly the surgical and respiratory medical units need access to high-risk equipment.

Decisions need to be made about whether or not to purchase or hire such equipment. Research carried out by one hospital (1988) estimated that a minimum of £15,000 per year could be saved if up-to-date preventative measures were implemented, and a further minimum of £10,000 could be saved by ensuring patients were identified at an early stage of being at risk of developing pressure sores.

Recommendations:

Immediate:
1. Replace all condemned mattresses with Transfoam mattresses. If they were replaced with the standard mattresses, this would be a false economy.
2. Each ward should draw up an action plan to deal with the individual problems identified in each area.
3. Discuss and agree the future provision of high-risk equipment.
4. Ensure that adequate lifting aids are available in each clinical area.

Long Term:
1. Half-yearly audits to monitor the number of pressure sores.
2. Undertake research into the prevention of pressure sores in cardio-thoracic patients.
3. Identify in future audits how many patients develop actual pressure sores following admission and how many patients are admitted with them.

References:

Bagust A 1992 Ward Nursing Quality and Grade Mix. York Health Economics Consortium, University of York, York.
Buchan J Ball J 1991 Caring Costs: Nursing Costs and Benefits. Institute of Manpower Studies, Brighton.
Department of Health 1991 The Patient's Charter. HMSO, London.
Hibbs P 1988 *Action against pressure sores.* Nursing Times 84, 13: 68-73.
Royal College of Nursing 1992 The Value of Nursing. RCN, London.
Waterlow, J. 1991 *A policy that protects* .Professional Nurse, Feb.: 258-264.

2 Continence Promotion

This case study illustrates how the setting and auditing of a standard highlighted the need for further resources and provided the staff with the information necessary to procure such resources to maintain specified outcomes. Nursing staff providing continuing care for the elderly developed a standard of care in order to improve the continence care they gave to their patients.

Over several weeks they reviewed the current relevant literature on continence needs of the elderly and sought advice from specialists such as the continence adviser. This helped them decide on the criteria that should be included in the standard and especially the outcomes they should be aiming for. Experience had shown them that elderly people admitted to hospital quickly developed difficulties with maintaining urinary continence. Some of the problems were related to physical causes such as constipation or restricted mobility, but other factors such as a change in environment, the stress of being away from home or family, or difficulties in communicating their needs to nursing staff also played their part.

The standard that resulted from their deliberations included process criteria, such as the nurse's assessment of continence needs of patients within 24 hours of admission, prompt responses to patients' requests for assistance in using toilet facilities and helping patients to select clothing according to patients' dexterity. Outcomes included the availability of a current assessment of continence needs and absence of regressive continence behaviour.

In accordance with usual practice the nurses devised an audit protocol/form in order to monitor their standard of care. This audit was carried out by members of the nursing team on a regular basis.

Unfortunately, during a period when there were several staff vacancies which had remained unfilled for some time, the results of their monitoring showed that the standard of care for continence promotion was not being maintained. In particular the nursing staff were able to identify that continence assessment was not being carried out within 24 hours of admission or at the time identified for reassessment. As a result there was evidence that the number of patients who developed regressive continence behaviours had increased.

Although the nurse manager had attempted to provide the ward with relief staff, they were often referred to as "pairs of hands". Many of the staff supplied were untrained or unfamiliar with continence needs of the elderly. In addition, they were unfamiliar with working practices developed to support the promotion of continence.

The senior nurse for practice development who had facilitated the nursing team in developing the standard collated the results of the monitoring and prepared a summary that showed the relationship between timely assessment by an experienced nurse and the number of patients developing regressive continence habits. This was then discussed with the Director of Nursing and nurse managers and as a result the staff vacancies were reviewed and arrangements made to fill the posts.

This experience demonstrates several important issues related to maintaining standards of patient care:

1. By developing the standard, nurses were able to define the relationship between the process of nursing and patient outcomes.

2. Standard setting had been a team exercise that represented shared values, professional experience and current knowledge, therefore the standard and resulting audit data were highly valued by the staff.

3. The nurse manager had access to clear, concise, objective information about the utilisation of resources and the subsequent effect on patient care.

4. After the standard had been developed, the nurse manager demonstrated her approval and support by endorsing the standard for both the process of care and the resources consumed.

The standard on continence promotion and the accompanying audit form are given below in Figures 2.2.1 and 2.2.2.

Figure 2.2.1 *Standard for Continence Promotion*

Topic	Individualised care	**Implement By Date**
Sub-Topic	Continence promotion	**Audit By Date**
Client Group	Elderly patients	**Head Signature**
Care Group		**Person Signature**
		Date
Standard Statement	Nursing care is organised to promote continence according to patient's individual requirements.	

STRUCTURE	PROCESS	OUTCOME
1. Toilets, commodes and accessories suitable for the elderly. Facilities for cleaning/disposal of toilet equipment.	1. The nurse participates in the selection of toileting equipment. The nurse ensures that toileting equipment is clean and ready for patient use.	1. Toileting arrangements meet the needs of the patient.
2. Toilets are clearly identified and consider the potential visual difficulties experienced by older people. Space between beds allows for the manoeuvring of commodes. Height adjustable beds. Unobstructed access to toilets. Good lighting. Working call bells and intercoms in all areas.	2. The nurse: – shows the patient the location of toilets; – demonstrates the use of call bells and intercoms; – checks the patient can operate them without difficulty; – answers call bells promptly.	2. The patient has immediate access to toilet facilities day and night.
3 Individual patient care plans. Information on continence promotion on ward. Continence adviser available. Post-basic courses on continence promotion.	3. Within 24 hours of admission and at identified intervals thereafter the nurse assesses the patient's continence needs including: – signs and behaviour used by the patient to communicate continence needs;	3. There is a current assessment of the patient's continence needs.

Figure 2.2.1 contd. *Standard for Continence Promotion*

Topic	Individualised care		Implement By Date
Sub-Topic	Continence promotion		Audit By Date
Client Group	Elderly patients		Head Signature
Care Group			Person Signature
			Date
Standard Statement	Nursing care is organised to promote continence according to patient's individual requirements.		

STRUCTURE	PROCESS	OUTCOME
4. A range of continence aids and products are on the ward.	4. The nurse plans and implements care including: – use of identified aids; – responding promptly to requests for assistance; – taking patients to toilet by shortest route; – encouraging mobility wherever possible; – identifying and responding to physical causes of incontinence at the earliest stage; – communicating patients' continence needs to other personnel.	4. The patient does not show regressive continence behaviour.
5. The ward housekeeper maintains patients' clothing.	5. The nurse assists the patient to select and wear clothing according to the patients' dexterity and continence needs.	5. The patient wears clothes which are clean and dry.

| – patterns/habits of continence; |
| – physical causes contributing to incontinence. |

104

Figure 2.2.2 *The Audit Protocol/form*

Sub-Topic: Continence promotion
Audit Objective: Nursing care promotes continence in elderly patients
Patient–Carer Sample: 3 randomly selected patients
Ward–Environment Sample: One early, late and night shift
Time-Frame: Per month
Auditors:
Date:

TARGET	METHOD	CODE	OUTCOME
Patient	Ask	2P	Do ambulant patients know where the nearest toilet is?
Patient	Ask	2P	Can the patient operate the call bell without difficulty or delay?
Patient	Ask	1O	Does the patient feel that the toilet facilities provided meet his requirements?
Nurses	Observe	2P	Does the nurse answer call bells promptly?
Nurses	Observe	3P	Does the nurse interpret patients' needs using established signs/language?
Nurses	Observe	4P	Does the nurse escort patients to the toilet without delay?
Ward equipment	Observe	2S	Is equipment used for toilet procedures clean and in good working order?
Ward equipment	Observe	1/2S	Is equipment used for toilet procedures suitable for elderly people?
Ward equipment	Observe	2S	Are routes to toilets unobstructed?
Care plan	Records	3P	Has an assessment of the patient's continence needs been made, according to standard, within 24 hours of admission?
Care plan	Records	3P	Has a time for reassessment of the patient's continence needs been identified?
Care plan	Records	4P	Does the care plan give precise directions as to how to meet the patient's continence needs?
Care plan	Records	4O	Is there evidence that the patient is showing regressive patterns of continence since admission to hospital?
Patients	Observe	5O	Does the patient's clothing require to be changed due to an incontinence problem?

3 The Lynebank Experience

This case study describes how one care setting responded to the challenge of quality improvement through standard setting activity. In particular it illustrates the evolving support structure which facilitated interprofessional activity within the hospital and highlights how the educational needs of staff were met.

The experience described took place in a hospital with 16 wards, a work therapy department, a recreational therapy department and a community nursing department. The hospital cares for people with learning difficulties and profound physical handicap.

In March 1987 four hospital-based charge nurses and two community charge nurses attended the initial area-wide study day for the introduction of standards of care. This study day was set up and facilitated by two clinical teachers and led by Alison Kitson, Project Co-ordinator for Standards of Care, Royal College of Nursing. Following this, all participants received the challenge to write standards from the Director of Nurse Education (DNE), with the offer of facilitation support and a second study day for consolidation.

The hospital took up the offer of support and a request was made for facilitation. This began with a meeting at which the charge nurses and one nurse manager were present. The concept of standard setting and some practicalities were discussed, further explanations were asked for and several points were clarified. The nurse manager was particularly interested in how she could assist in the development. Two draft standards were discussed with a view to presenting these at the follow-up study day planned for three months later. This group, including the newly interested nurse manager, was to attend the second study day.

Following the second study day the two clinical teachers, who by now had been allocated time by the DNE for facilitation, met with the Director of Nursing Services who was interested to know more so he could support this initiative. A decision was made for the facilitators to make a presentation to all senior nursing staff on standard setting.

The reception from the senior nursing staff was mixed, as they were fairly unsure of their role in this venture, but nonetheless the general attitude was very supportive. It was agreed that the facilitators would carry out teaching sessions within the hospital on "An Introduction to Standard Setting" with a view to all nursing staff becoming involved in the initiative.

Ward Staff are Introduced to Standard Setting

Sessions set up included four afternoon workshops for trained and untrained day staff, two evening sessions for night staff and one session for community staff.

There was a high degree of commitment by senior nurses and the "already involved" nurse manager to these workshops and no half-days were taken by staff on these days to enable everyone to attend the sessions during the autumn of 1987. The workshops had been arranged so that each grade of staff attended with their peers.

The nurse manager attended each workshop, introducing herself and the facilitators to the groups at the beginning of each session and, at the end, challenged the staff to produce a standard within a reasonable period of time – approximately six weeks. My initial reaction to the direct challenge and the time limit given was "Is this right? – It's very directive, will it work?"

The general response from staff seemed positive at the sessions although, at the first one for staff nurses, many were fairly quiet and appeared demoralised. There was neither debate nor overt negativity and as the workshop progressed enthusiasm increased and a willingness to participate was demonstrated.

To keep the standard setting profile high I suggested that standard setting should be itemised on already established agendas for ward meetings and senior nurse meetings – hoping that in time, as work increased, meetings would develop for standard setting activities alone.

The Response to Introductory Sessions

Following the nurse manager's suggestion to write a standard, each ward formed a standard setting group which identified an area for quality improvement within each ward, gathered the information necessary and developed a standard. As this work progressed the nurse manager and facilitators agreed it would be a good idea for the facilitators to visit each ward and discuss their progress on standard writing to give them encouragement and advice.

A programme was devised by one of the two senior nurses within the hospital for the facilitators to spend 30 minutes in each ward and department over a period of two days. These sessions quickly became known as "walkabouts". The programme, although originally planned for a two-day period was adapted and extended over a three-week period as it became apparent that the staff needed more than 30 minutes. Each session took one hour with staff attending from night duty and days off. A variety of issues was addressed at such sessions.

Many nurses wanted to discuss the identity and future of nursing in general, while others were concerned with internal politics. During the walkabouts we were given several labels including "helpers", "listeners", and even "spies from the Health Board".

On visiting recreational therapy and work therapy, staff identified the need to know about standard setting, particularly those workers within the departments who had not had any previous information on standard setting. They were interested and wanted to know more, so on the walkabout a mini seminar with overheads and examples was held to clarify their ideas. In care settings where standards were being developed, assistance was needed to refine their subject to a more manageable size before they could identify criteria.

Many different care issues were being explored, and out of these, three standard setting ward teams identified personalised clothing as an issue for quality improvement. This could have been seen as duplication, and two wards could have been guided to find an alternative. In allowing them all to continue to work on this issue, however, a number of benefits ensued. Many criteria were identified, taking account of the differing needs of the client groups within the three wards; in addition the staff learned the process of standard setting by choosing to work on an aspect of care they felt strongly about; finally the hospital management team was being alerted to an area of care which needed priority attention.

Other wards were writing standards which required consultation or negotiation with nurse managers or other disciplines before they could be implemented, therefore the staff wanted advice on how to go about taking this action.

By the end of January 1988 the first round of walkabouts was completed by one of the two facilitators and thereafter discussions on progress took place with the senior nurses. Some of the standards were now ready for typing and signing. With regard to the groups, some needed further assistance with refining, while others needed management support to enable changes to take place.

I suggested that monthly unit meetings be set up for exchange, sharing and support so that staff had ongoing regular support and assistance. A representative from each ward attended this meeting along with her nurse manager, the clinical teacher and the already interested nurse manager, who were now both emerging as local facilitators for the staff. Around this time the two key facilitators were visited by Hannie Giebing, Project Co-ordinator, Nursing Quality Assurance, National Organization for Quality Assurance (The Netherlands) who confirmed this arrangement for support and communication, as it was already in place and working successfully within the organisation in The Netherlands.

A request then came from the hospital management team for a seminar on standard setting. Those who participated were the support services manager, domestic services manager, works manager, hospital manager, psychologist and doctor. The team had been asked to write "Quality Standards" by their unit general manager. A previous attempt had been made by administrative staff to define "standards", but on seeing what the nurses were doing they decided to scrap existing work and learn about the Dynamic Standard Setting System. This was emphasised particularly by the support services manager.

Development of Support Structure

The next step was to consider hospital co-ordination of the activities and promote interprofessional working.

Communication increased between the local facilitators and the support services manager as she sought advice on standard setting and refining criteria. At this time the standards written by nursing staff on personalised clothing had implications for sewing-room and laundry services. It became apparent that co-operation from these departments would enhance these standards.

Because the hospital management team was interested and there was an obvious need for interprofessional collaboration to fully implement the standards, it seemed an ideal time to set up a hospital co-ordinating group. In the first instance, I thought this group would consist of senior nurses who would link into the hospital management team for decision-making. It was agreed, however, that this group should be interprofessional. The membership and function of the group were discussed. All disciplines were represented on the group including the clinical teacher of the hospital who was now functioning as a facilitator working in partnership with the nurse manager. Representation included senior nurse manager, facilitator nurse manager, facilitator clinical teacher, works officer, psychologist, doctor, support services manager, physiotherapist, and myself as key facilitator.

This group took on the function already outlined in Part One Chapter Four, with the additional function of acting as a forum for negotiating change. This became a natural development because of the interprofessional nature of the group.

All standards which appeared to have implications for other disciplines were discussed by this group with regard to how they should be implemented. Initially it was extremely difficult to stick to discussing only those criteria and not go off on a tangent by rewriting all the criteria. We had to remind ourselves that changing the standards was not the responsibility of the group. Since nurses had led the project, all standards developed in the first few months were nursing standards. However, there were soon requests for the local facilitators to spend time clarifying issues with paramedical staff and assist them in writing standards. Meeting monthly at the co-ordinating group facilitated such invitations.

By spring 1988, approximately 20 standards were in operation. Sub-topics covered at this point included personalised clothing, well-fitting footwear, daily communication among staff and maintenance of privacy. The nurse manager and clinical teacher continued as a team, facilitating ward groups to meet, develop standards, refine criteria and make changes.

About this time an area-wide two-day workshop for local facilitators was set up which further equipped the nurse manager for her role. She spoke at the workshop on some of her experiences as a facilitator, being well ahead of other areas represented in setting up the system. By this time there was only one key facilitator, but she was in a substantive full-time post and fulfilling the remit described for key facilitator in Part One Chapter Five.

Sustaining the Effort – Highlights and Challenges

Ongoing education has always been a priority within this hospital, and was identified as such by the local facilitators whenever the need arose. The next venture was to be an interprofessional half-day workshop. Eight nursing staff and eight support service staff were represented – including domestic, catering, administrative and portering. This afternoon session was led by myself (as key facilitator) and assisted by the two local facilitators. An offshoot of this study afternoon involved the head porter in writing a standard which was to alter the mortuary environment, initiate training in sensitivity for the porters when escorting bereaved relatives to the mortuary and change the face of standard setting to an even more interprofessional approach.

The next step was to hold an area-wide study day on monitoring standards, and this hospital was represented by various members of staff including the support services manager who, by this time, was actively facilitating support services in standard setting. Before venturing into monitoring standards within the hospital I made a request to the facilitator that each ward team write a few lines to answer the following questions:
"Why did you write the standard?"
"What changes have you made as a result?"
Both the facilitators and myself were pleasantly surprised that the "few lines" became pages and demonstrated a positive staff attitude to standards and the changes made as a result of standard setting activities.

The time had now come for all wards to set about monitoring their standards, yet only a few had attended the study day, so a half-day workshop was set up within the hospital. All wards were represented to work on devising a monitoring tool for their standard. The request then came from support services to do likewise. A half-day workshop was set up, and all domestic and administrative services, clothing manager, catering and sewing-room staff members were represented. This particular afternoon was a very special experience for me as the sewing-room staff member read out her standard and monitoring tool on "measuring male residents accurately for well-fitting trousers". The discussion which followed was fascinating and the points which arose were as follows:
– the need for accurate and consistent measurement of the men
– documentation of a person's measurement, i.e. who should measure
– where and how this should be done
– where and when it should be documented
– deformity/physical handicap needed to be taken into consideration.

To date, nurses had done much of the measuring, resulting sometimes in inaccuracy and inconsistency. An example was cited where nurses were observed trying to measure the person while he remained seated. This standard now had implications for *nurses.* So the tables were turned. The group was moving upward in the spiral to improve quality.

As time moved on we were challenged as key and local facilitators when several trained staff moved from one particular ward where they had been working with a standard on therapeutic play. The new charge nurse and staff nurse did not agree with the standard.

When this was discussed with me I wondered "What are they really saying here? Is it a question of ownership, or is it an unrealistic standard? Was it being met before?" It certainly could not just be scrapped and another written to replace it. I suggested that before any changes were made they should monitor the standard. Following this it was then agreed to alter one of the criteria, as the time of day identified within the standard for the activity was not particularly suitable. This experience raised the question of ownership of the standard, realistic standards and the need for close support from facilitators.

Around the same time, staff numbers decreased on this ward and this caused further frustration and dissatisfaction among the remaining staff as they could not meet even the reviewed standard. Following a meeting between key and local facilitators and hospital manager to explain what was happening, the hospital manager agreed to discuss concerns with the staff. On this occasion the standard acted as a valuable basis for discussion and the result was a more enlightened hospital manager, who shared the responsibility of not being able to meet the standard at this time and took time to discuss this with the ward staff.

One new charge nurse at the hospital thought standard setting was a paper exercise and a waste of time. During his induction he was directed to the Philosophy of Nursing and Health Board Core Standards. He challenged these, and in particular: *Every patient/client/resident in hospital receives nursing care in an optimal therapeutic environment.* He used the standard to write a paper with recommendations to draw attention to the changes to be made for his ward to meet these criteria. Subsequently this was discussed with the local and key facilitators and a realistic plan was proposed. The result was a much-changed ward environment – a more homely decoration with partitions erected for privacy between bath and shower, plants, pictures and festoon blinds on an internal window. In this way an area-wide core standard was used to enable a positive change in the environment. He was less negative after this experience.

The winter of 1989 witnessed an extensive monitoring exercise led by the local facilitator (nurse manager) and guided by the key facilitator. Monitoring tools had been developed by staff and vetted by the facilitators for all standards.

Following the monitoring activity which was carried out by the ward teams themselves, the results were sent to the local facilitator. She in turn analysed the data and discussed with the ward teams the problems, successes and priorities following monitoring, the action to be taken and a new date for monitoring. This activity was followed up by a visit to the wards by the key facilitator to discuss issues, problems and successes and to reinforce support to the local facilitator.

Although within this specialty residents are moving into the community, future staff posts are uncertain and morale at times is low, standards activity continues. One comment from an enrolled nurse recently was "We keep going because support is always there. Our queries are always answered."

By spring 1990 the hospital had approximately 60 standards including sewing room, portering, domestic services, physiotherapy, nursing and interprofessional standards (Howell and Marr 1988,Marr and Pirie 1990). One of the more recent initiatives was a joint medical, nursing and pharmaceutical standard.

In many ways this particular hospital led the way in setting up a durable support structure and a forum for negotiating change. There was of course the usual lip service, sabotage and inertia. On the other hand, however, there was also motivation and committed people who supported attitude and behaviour change to improve the quality of care and quality of life for those residents with learning difficulties.

Heather Marr
Fife 1990

References:

Howell J and Marr H (1988) *Visible improvements* Nursing Times Vol. 84 (25): 33-34.
Marr H and Pirie M (1990) *Protecting privacy* Nursing Times Vol. 86 (13): 58-59.

4 The Development of Two Local Standards

This chapter provides examples of the development of two standards, one as a case study, the second as a flow chart. The first standard is concerned with the tragic circumstances surrounding the experience of cot death and a hospital staff's response to this in a quality improvement activity. The second example addresses the very important issue of patient education. It is interesting to note in the first example that the changes were implemented because of the writing of the standard, whereas in the second, the standard (Figure 2.3.2) was written after the changes had been made, in order to maintain the improved quality in patient education.

Sudden Infant Death
This case study describes how a standard setting group put into practice their ideas for improvement in care (Addison, 1990). As a result they were able to make major changes in the care given to parents and family following cot death. After facilitating a series of workshops on standard setting within a hospital providing accident and emergency services, outpatient services and surgical care, each ward and department set about identifying an area for quality improvement. As the key facilitator, I was invited to visit the accident and emergency department to attend a quality improvement meeting at which the care given to parents following cot death was discussed. It was agreed that the group would meet at a time most suiting their work commitment and that the meeting should last no more than one and a half hours. The group consisted of three charge nurses (one from night duty), three first level and two second level nurses.

In order to focus on a manageable and defined project I asked the group why they had chosen this subject. I expected that the reasons they would identify would become the issues for quality improvement. The reason given for the choice, however, was that the Director of Nursing Services had in fact chosen that particular area of care for the group. With this in mind we backtracked to discuss the group's feelings about someone else identifying the subject for them. Although short, this discussion was very productive.

At the outset of the discussion, commitment to this subject was varied with other concerns in the participants' minds apart from this one. However, once the group members realised that the subject chosen was not just an idea plucked out of the air but was part of a wider initiative, they then became committed to the issue and were all agreed in taking this particular idea forward.

The next step for the group was to discuss what the current procedure was for dealing with the situation and the discussion was concerned with examples and incidents from the individual experiences of the members. At the same time the group discussed why they were carrying out care in this way and suggestions were made for improvement. All the ideas which were forthcoming at this stage were written down by the facilitator. Following this part of the discussion, the key quality theme which was emerging was *Dignity and Support.* This theme became the focus for the group and a draft standard statement was developed which embraced this theme (Figure 2.4.1).

In a relatively short time the group reached agreement about the kind of care which ought to be given to bereaved parents and families and the changes which had to be made in order to achieve this. The discussion highlighted a number of current issues which the staff were unhappy with, including the equipment used, the inadequate information they sometimes received from the police and the environment within which counselling took place. This gathering of information and discussion took around one hour. The next task was to identify the impact of this on the client. This, together with the suggestions for improvement, now formed the basis for the structure, process and outcome criteria.

Because of the enthusiasm in the group, the information gathered at the meeting was formulated into criteria quickly. Within two days the team were implementing the changes, including negotiating for a partitioned room within the accident and emergency department where parents could be met with in a more dignified environment. Within a month the activity had hospital management support, including financial support. The room was furnished, the guidelines were adapted to suit the local conditions and the articles identified in the structure criteria were bought. Although the negotiations with the police were more difficult, as a result of a two-hour discussion with them about the changes needed, agreement was finally reached. As a result of all of this, a tragic situation would now be less traumatic for parents and staff.

Auditing of the standard happened naturally and quickly after the implementation of the standard. Following each cot death incident within the department the staff held a post-care meeting to discuss whether the criteria had been met, and if not, why not. The discussion at the meetings centred on the actual practice and responses from the parents themselves or from the health visitor carrying out bereavement visits. Feedback often came in the form of a letter/card from parents or subsequent visits to the department with other children. A detailed report with the findings of the meeting was then written, and any action needed to refine the standard was taken.

Two examples of criteria which were altered as a result of incidents which actually took place are as follows:

Figure 2.4.1 *Standard for Sudden Infant Death*

Topic	Individualised Care	**Achieve Standard by**
Sub-Topic	Dignity and Support	**Review Standard by**
Care Group	Parents and Family Following Cot Death	**Signature of DNS**
		Signature of Senior Nurse
Standard Statement	Sudden Infant Death Syndrome babies will be treated with dignity and the parents' needs met as identified.	

STRUCTURE	PROCESS	OUTCOME
1. Staff are notified of all Sudden Infant Death Syndrome babies sent to the mortuary by ambulance depot and police.	1. Skilled nurse; one designated by the senior nurse as having the skill to deal with the situation.	1. Relatives arriving either with, or to view, a baby are met immediately on arrival.
2. A Moses basket, clothes and shawl are available.	2. Privacy from others is arranged.	2. A private room is arranged and a nurse delegated to escort the clients and remain with them.
3. A private room for clients.	3. Present the baby with loving care in as natural a climate as possible.	3. Assessment of clients needs are acted on by nurse escort.
4. A room outwith the mortuary is available to see baby.	4. Assess the needs, physical and mental and necessary support required.	4. Seeing baby for the last time is done in acceptable and dignified conditions without haste.
5. Procedure guidelines are available.	5. Notify clergy, priest or relative re support.	5. Photographs are taken if desired for parents.
6. Information for reading: Information on Sudden Infant Death Syndrome and Parents' Reaction and Fear. List of telephone numbers: Police (Local) Ambulance Health Visitor	6. Allow parents as much time as they wish.	6. All support by family or back up services is dealt with and recorded.
	7. Arrange transport and confirm home reception suitable.	7. Records made of call to health visitors.
	8. Nurse co-ordinates support service back up, by phoning health visitors and recording call.	

- baby clothes of varying sizes
- the introduction of a camera and taking of photographs of the baby with the parents' permission.

Since I facilitated the group in the writing of this standard, I frequently use it as an example when teaching standard setting, in order to highlight the major changes accomplished by staff at the grass roots. It is now the case that many hospitals are implementing this standard. Even modern purpose-built hospitals where no problem was perceived have examined closely their practice and the environment where such care is carried out, and subsequently similar changes are being made.

Because the staff developed the standard and therefore have ownership of it they have the responsibility to implement, monitor and review it. It seems to me that this dynamic process of continuous improvement would not take place if the standard had been sent to the participants by someone outwith the department, or alternatively if a room had just been created within the department as a result of a management initiative.

To ensure the ongoing high-quality care within this standard the importance of the following cannot be underestimated:
- the post-care meeting which facilitates peer group review
- the sensitivity with which the standard was adjusted and finely tuned
  in response to needs identified by parents and relatives at this
  extremely painful time
- the effect of being able to examine the collated reports retrospectively,
  and visually present these findings to a quality assurance committee
- the previously outlined positive effects of the participation and involvement of
  staff, increasing commitment to any subsequent changes.

Heather Marr
Fife

Patient Education
The following example outlines how patient education was tackled in a hospital caring for people with chest disorders. It had been noted in this particular hospital that patients were sometimes being discharged without a sound knowledge of their condition and often without written information about the changes needed to promote a healthier lifestyle (Figure 2.4.2).

The Health Promotion Department was tasked with the responsibility of identifying the extent of the problem and of devising an action plan to remedy the situation. In this quality improvement activity, the flow chart (Figure 2.4.3) is used to demonstrate the progress from the recognition of the problem to its resolution in a concise and comprehensive manner.

Figure 2.4.2 *Standard for Patient Education*

Topic	Health Education	Achieve Standard by
Sub-Topic	Availability of Information	Review Standard by
Care Group	All Patients/clients in Chest Unit	Signature of DNS
Source of Production	Chest Unit	Signature of Senior Nurse
Standard Statement	Individual patients are kept fully informed about all aspects of health education pertaining to his/her condition and can demonstrate this knowledge.	

STRUCTURE	PROCESS	OUTCOME
The nurse has the knowledge and skills to assess, plan, implement and evaluate a patient education programme.	The nurse listens to the patient and assesses the extent of his/her knowledge and concerns.	The patient demonstrates a clear understanding, either practically or verbally, of the information/education given to him/her.
This will cover knowledge of the:- 1. patient's condition/illness 2. patient's treatment 3. prognosis 4. educational programme	The nurse documents the findings on the appropriate check list.	The nurse documents the outcome of the educational programme.
In order to develop the necessary skills for effective patient education, the nurse has the opportunity to attend relevant courses on communication skills, counselling and health education.	The nurse, with the patient, must identify and prioritise the individual learning needs of the patient. The nurse plans and documents the agreed educational programme.	
	Using the appropriate teaching methods and resources, the nurse helps the patient fulfil the agreed plan.	
	The nurse documents this process.	
	The nurse refers the patient to other members of the multidisciplinary team, eg: dietician, physiotherapist, where appropriate.	

Figure 2.4.3 *Patient Education Flowchart*

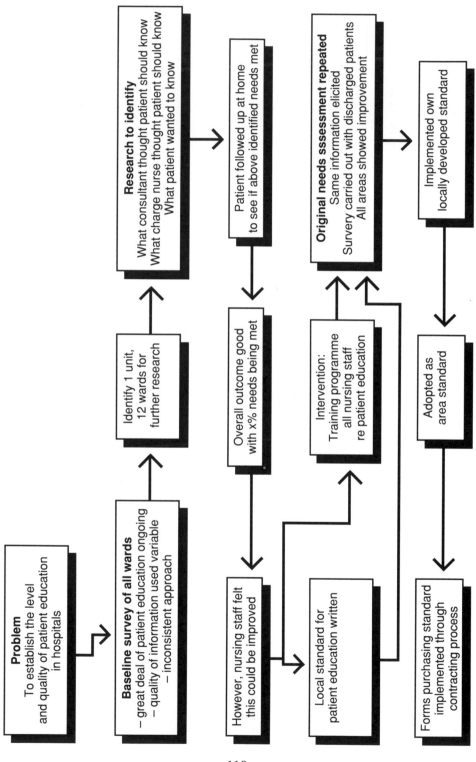

Problem
To establish the level
and quality of patient education
in hospitals

Baseline survey of all wards
– great deal of patient education ongoing
– quality of information used variable
– inconsistent approach

Identify 1 unit,
12 wards for
further research

Research to identify
What consultant thought patient should know
What charge nurse thought patient should know
What patient wanted to know

Patient followed up at home
to see if above identified needs met

Overall outcome good
with x% needs being met

However, nursing staff felt
this could be improved

Local standard for
patient education written

Intervention:
Training programme
all nursing staff
re patient education

Original needs sssessment repeated
Same information elicited
Survery carried out with discharged patients
All areas showed improvement

Implemented own
locally developed standard

Adopted as
area standard

Forms purchasing standard
implemented through
contracting process

The key points to note in this example are:
- the standard grew out of a research needs assessment
- it was a collaborative venture (nursing and health promotion staff)
- it was part of an audit cycle
- the standard developed from local → area → purchasing standard. The standard began as a local standard implemented firstly in the wards chosen for further research. It then progressed to area level where it was implemented throughout the health board. In the more recent purchaser–provider relationship it has been specified as a standard to be met by providers within the purchasing specification.

References

Addison W 1990 *Setting standards of compassion.* Nursing Standard ,January 24 Vol. 4 No. 18 22-24.

5 Moving and Handling

This case study focuses on how a standard adapted for a particular care setting was audited. The process of checking how the standard was being met highlighted areas of good practice and areas requiring attention, some of which were within the standard setting group's responsibility, others being the responsibility of management.

In the early days of standard setting, three members of staff from Fife College of Nursing and Midwifery interested in standard setting paid a two-day visit to West Berkshire Health Authority to learn of the developments made primarily by Helen Kendall. From that visit, Fife's Director of Nurse Education and two clinical teachers were to become enthused by such beginnings.

Following the visit, there was a desire and a commitment to set up a similar project within Fife Health Board. Examples were given as to how such a system could improve the practice of nursing. One such example has stood the test of time and has been used extensively to teach standard setting. Not only has it been used to teach, but in addition a large number of nurses have embraced it as their own, adopting or adapting it to their own situation. The standard is concerned with *moving and handling*, an issue of prime concern to professionals and managers. This standard was adapted for clients being cared for in the community by a standard setting group of district nursing sisters and was then audited to check if the standard was being met.

The audit took the form of questionnaires for clients, carers and staff.

The Questionnaires

150 nurses on both day and " tucking down" duty, including qualified nurses and nursing assistants, returned their questionnaires. The collated findings are given in Figure 2.5.1. Numbers did not permit the inclusion of every client and carer on the district nurses' caseloads, therefore one patient and his or her carer (if there was one) from each district nurse's caseload was chosen. The questionnaires (Figures 2.5.2 & 2.5.3) were answered by clients and carers who were randomly selected by a delegated peer. 56 clients and 48 carers were used in the sample. This questionnaire will be changed for future use to ensure that previously recorded injuries are not included.

Figure 2.5.1 *The Nurse Questionnaire*

Question	Yes	No	Remarks
1. Have you received training in the principles of kinetic movement?	139 93%	11 7%	Update requested by some.
2. Are mechanical aids available to you when required?	83 55%	67 45%	Occasionally unavailable. Delayed delivery. Not always. Sometimes waiting list.
3. Are you trained to use the mechanical aids provided?	93 62%	57 38%	No formal training. Sometimes no instructions with aid. Rep or physiotherapist consulted by individual nurses. Nurses train each other.
4. Are written instructions supplied with the mechanical aid?	47 31%	103 69%	Sometimes. Depends on equipment. Not always.
5. Are you aware of Health and Safety policy on lifting?	126 84%	24 16%	Not able to find policy.
6. Does the district nursing sister perform the initial assessment for the aid?	144 96%	6 4%	Depends on staffing levels.
7. Are the special lifting needs/aids recorded in the patients' records?	132 88%	18 12%	Yes, but requires regular updating. Not always. Don't know. (1)
8. Is suitably trained assistance available to you?	95 63%	55 37%	Not always – staffing levels – geography of area – sickness – weekends & emergency situations.
9. Does the patient receive a full explanation of lifting technique?	146 97%	4 3%	If applicable – desirable – relevant. Routinely.
10. Is the lifting technique for each individual patient consistent?	123 82%	27 18%	May be differences between nurses. Difficult to assess due to number of carers involved.
11. Does the district nursing sister evaluate the care plan regularly?	145 97%	5 3%	No comments.
12. Does the district nursing sister consult with staff involved?	143 95%	7 5%	No comments.

Figure 2.5.1 contd. *The Nurse Questionnaire*

Question	Yes	No	Remarks
13. Have you sustained any injury related to lifting in the last year? (If yes please give details in remarks column)	14 9%	136 91%	Family reluctant to have equipment. Emergency situation. Twisting of joint or spinal column (10 weeks sick). X-ray taken. (1) 2 nurses – injuries caused by same patient. Hoist now installed.

Figure 2.5.2 *The Client Questionnaire*

Question	Yes	No	Remarks
1. Has a full explanation of the lifting technique been given to you?	47 84%	9 16%	Patient's co-ordination, concentration and memory poor. Electric hoist used by nurses.
2. Do all staff lift in the manner explained to you?	49 87%	7 13%	Nursing staff do but not untrained staff.
3. Do you feel secure and comfortable when being lifted?	51 91%	5 9%	It's not the lifting that hurts but the arthritis. Panic is a problem. Patient nervous of hoist.
4. Have you sustained any injury during lifting?	9 16%	47 84%	Patients have been injured when lifted by relatives.

Figure 2.5.3 *The Carer Questionnaire*

Question	Yes	No	Remarks
1. Has the nurse explained the lifting technique to you?	41 85%	7 15%	Engineer who fitted two hoists explained technique
2. Has the technique been demonstrated to you?	43 90%	5 10%	Not involved in lifting.
3. Do you feel confident to carry out this procedure?	43 90%	5 10%	Unable to help now. As long as someone else can help. Own method of lifting – no problem.
4. Have you sustained any injury while lifting?	24 50%	24 50%	Shoulder strain. Back injury. Back ache.
5. Does the district nursing sister communicate any change in technique to you?	42 88%	6 12%	

The following are the key issues and actions which emerged, after the results of the audit had been presented to management.

Nurse questionnaire

Question 2 — Are mechanical aids available to you when required?
Problem — The lack of mechanical aids available was highlighted.
Action — The Community Care service strategy will endeavour to meet increased requirements for equipment. Additional funds are to be made available through service planning, transfers of funding and reallocation of resources.

Question 4 — Are written instructions supplied with the mechanical aid?
Problem — Lack of written instructions supplied with aid.
Action — Supplier clinic was contacted and requested to include written instructions when delivering equipment.

Carer questionnaire

Question 4 — Have you sustained any injury while lifting?
Problem — High rate of injury identified.
Action — The Community Care service strategy should include as a key task for 1991-93, the development of a training programme on moving and handling techniques for staff.

Carer & Client Questionnaire

Question 4 (in both) — Have you sustained any injury while lifting?
Problem — Need for rewording of one question.
Action — The Carer & Client questionnaire will have to be reworded to ensure that previously recorded injuries are not included in subsequent audits.

The Health and Safety Executive has identified in a guidance note that approximately 25% of all occupational injuries reported can be attributed to handling of loads including persons. From available statistics the most at-risk groups include nurses, porters and ambulance crews. It is therefore important that this particular standard (Figure 2.5.4) is implemented thoroughly and monitored regularly.

Implementation of the standard has highlighted areas of good practice and areas of deficiency which have assisted in identifying areas of priority. It is hoped that subsequent monitoring and audit will indicate a reducing trend in the number of lifting-related injuries.

Figure 2.5.4 *Standard for Moving and Handling*

Topic:	Safety
Sub Topic:	Moving and Handling
Standard Statement:	Moving and handling is carried out in a manner which protects patients and staff from injury

6 The Development of Management Standards in Nursing

This case study outlines how concern to meet objectives within the *Strategy for Nursing, Midwifery and Health Visiting* prompted a group of nurse managers to develop standards and audit forms for use within one organisation.

Although standards were being set nationally about issues of clinical care and the wider service, few standards were addressing the framework and culture within which people were having to work. Certainly within one health board where standards of care had been developed for some time, nurse managers agreed it was time to develop a philosophy of management in nursing, midwifery and health visiting and core management standards. Furthermore, following the introduction of the *Strategy for Nursing, Midwifery and Health Visiting* (1990), it was highlighted that although many of the objectives identified within practice, education, management and research were being taken forward, issues concerning management standards had not yet been dealt with. It was agreed by nurses in management that the development of management standards would progress the following objectives from the strategy.

- "Nursing resources need to be deployed effectively and efficiently. The White Paper on the NHS, *Working for Patients* makes it clear that this is crucial if the objectives for the Health Service in Scotland are to be attained. To achieve it, managers and nurses need an agreed framework within which to work. Such a framework must reflect the purpose and philosophy of professional nursing and recognise the contribution of nursing services to health care." (1.1)
- "To contribute to effective manpower planning including issues such as skill mix and deployment which takes account of strategic plans, standards to be met, and available resources." (5.2.2)
- "To operate an effective system for appraisal and development of staff, including the identification and planned development of those showing leadership potential." (5.2.3)

The following is a description of the preparatory work involved. In response to these concerns, a background paper was written and circulated by the key facilitator of standards of care within the organisation. This paper was to form the basis for the development of management standards. The background paper was written to promote discussion and subsequent action among all middle and senior managers and was based on the document *Standards of Care Management in Nursing* (RCN, 1989) recently published at that time.

The paper outlined the suggested content for a philosophy of management in nursing (Figure 2.6.1) and developed key themes in nursing management, emphasising at the outset that: "It is important to distinguish between managing nursing and managing nurses. We believe that only nurses can manage nursing." (op. cit.)

Figure 2.6.1 *Philosophy of Management in Nursing, Midwifery and Health Visiting*

---

*Nursing Management is an integral part of the general management framework and provides the structure within which nurses work.

Nurses in management are committed to:

achieving excellence and providing a quality service

creating the organisational framework which enables the effective and efficient promotion of health and provision of holistic care for the patient/client and his family

quality being a key element built into every process within the organisation through standard setting and monitoring to achieve excellence in client centred care

a sensitivity to the welfare and development of staff, considering their health, safety and well-being

creating a climate of trust and respect enabling involvement in decision making and creativity

utilising resources in a creative and fair way

the development of relevant and accurate information systems and timely and meaningful operational policies

equipping staff to practise in accordance with the UKCC Code of Professional Conduct

enabling the implementation of the *Strategy for Nursing, Midwifery and Health Visiting* in Scotland (1990)

The above gives a clarity of purpose with stated values to provide an effective organisation in which staff can grow.

Nurses in management aim to enable those who work in the service to:

achieve its purpose

share its values

feel valued themselves

*To avoid repetition, the terms 'nurse' and 'nursing' are generally used in the text to refer to the three professions of nursing, midwifery and health visiting.

Within the published document (RCN, 1989), each of the key themes identified was subdivided into a number of standard statements. The key themes outlined in the discussion paper were as follows:
– philosophy and objectives
– organisation and management
– managing resources – human
– managing resources – financial
– policies and procedures
– management of care
– quality assurance and evaluation.

In the discussion paper it was suggested that core standards be identified from the themes. These broad standards could then be adopted or adapted locally to relate more specifically to organisational frameworks, geographical areas and service priorities. It was appreciated that the standards would have varying relevance for managers depending on their role and function within the organisation.

Following distribution of the background paper, a working party was set up to work together to develop the philosophy, core standards and audit forms within a six-month period. During the development process, colleagues were consulted informally and then a draft document was formally circulated for consultation to all nurses in management.

The seven standards which were developed by the group are given in Figures 2.6.2 to 2.6.8. It can be seen that the standard on the interview process (Figure 2.6.8) had already been written by the personnel department and was adapted by the group.

At least the following three recommendations can be made to maximise the implementation of these standards.
1. Refine or adapt the standards for your area of responsibility/department/locality.
2. Develop audit forms and carry out an audit to find out what is happening at the moment in your area.
3. Discuss the standards with managers outwith nursing and develop the philosophy and standards on an interprofessional basis.

Figure 2.6.2 *Standard for Statutory Requirements*

Topic/Sub-Topic	Professional Accountability/U.K.C.C. Code of Professional Conduct	Review Standard by
Client Group	Nursing Staff	**Signature of CANO**
Ref	Nurses in Management	**Date**
Standard Statement	Nurse management has systems in place to ensure that staff are equipped to practise in accordance with U.K.C.C. Code of Professional Conduct	
Rationale	Nurse managers must ensure that local policies and procedures are based upon U.K.C.C. documentation	

STRUCTURE	PROCESS	OUTCOME
All current U.K.C.C. documentation is accessible to staff Code of Professional Conduct 3rd ed. (1992) Exercising Accountability (1989) Confidentiality (1987) The Scope of Professional Practice (1992) A Guide for Students of Nursing & Midwifery (1992) All current Health Board policies and procedures are available to staff at all levels Grievance procedure and disciplinary procedure are available in all wards and departments	Nurses in management: provide information to in-service/continuing education departments on new skills/knowledge required have a responsibility to set up and maintain induction, orientation and appraisal programmes within their area are responsible for checking that all nurses' registration with U.K.C.C. is current and accurate facilitate the use and accessibility to U.K.C.C. documentation with all staff within their responsibility monitor that staff comply with the Code of Conduct to provide acceptable levels of care handle grievance procedure in accordance with Health Board procedure give reward and recognition apply and implement disciplinary procedure ensure that Health Board policies are accessible and current	A recognised staff/service development programme is in place Individual appraisal takes place according to programme Staff practice within their grade and job description Staff act in a professional manner Staff deliver a competent service Staff recognise and honour direct and indirect accountability borne for all aspects of professional practice (see 9.5 The Scope of Professional Practice)

Figure 2.6.3 *Standard for Appraisal System*

Topic/Sub-Topic	Personnel/Staff Appraisal	**Review Standard by**
		Signature of CANO
		Date
Client Group	Nursing Staff	
Ref	Nurses in Management	
Standard Statement	All staff are facilitated to participate in an effective appraisal system which reviews job performance	
Rationale	Staff are entitled to an annual appraisal to identify attributes and limitations, exchange ideas and plan future objectives	

STRUCTURE	PROCESS	OUTCOME
Current appraisal documentation	Nurses in management:	Enhanced staff performance
An ongoing programme for staff members	set up appraisal interview as a formal appointment with staff member	Exchange of ideas between staff member and manager
Uninterrupted time/quiet private room	assess and review job performance	Staff appraisal goals are met
	use interview to highlight achievements, review existing objectives and agree new objectives	A sense of achievement by each staff member
	review objectives 6 monthly	
	facilitate the expression of concerns	
	identify and agree training needs	
	promote self-assessment	

Figure 2.6.4 *Standard for Staff Development*

Topic/Sub-Topic	Personnel/Professional and Personal Development	Review Standard by
Client Group	Nursing Staff	Signature of CANO
Ref	Nurses in Management	Date
Standard Statement	Staff have the opportunity to participate in a professional and personal programme promoting optimal development within the needs and confines of the service	
Rationale	Staff must endeavour to achieve, maintain and develop knowledge, skill and competence to respond to the needs and interests of patients.	

STRUCTURE	PROCESS	OUTCOME
Nurses in management have a knowledge of: a) existing programmes b) new developments making demands on in-service training c) statutory requirements The Scope of Professional Practice (1992) P.R.E.P. (1992) d) budget allocation for training Course information is available ahead of time Formal liaison systems exist with personnel, continuing education and in-service departments	Nurses in management: identify requirements in advance nominate for courses based on staff appraisal, availability, interest, specialty and fairness contact buget holder for authorisation complete necessary documentation for application ensure staff are briefed prior to course ensure maintenance of service provision in absence set up feedback and evaluation of course ensure that nurses are assisted to undertake any adjustment to their scope of practice	Identified staff development needs are documented and retained by nurse manager Prioritised service and staff development Individual potential in maximised Detailed information of attendance at courses is held by individual record/profile/centrally

Figure 2.6.5 *Standard for Communication Systems*

Topic/Sub-Topic	Management/Communication Systems	Review Standard by
Client Group	Nursing Staff	**Signature of CANO**
Ref	Nurses in Management	**Date**
Standard Statement	Effective two way communication systems are developed and maintained at all levels within the organisation which are practical, achievable, facilitate two way communication and promote action	
Rationale	Essential to the overall management of the nursing service is the ease with which nurses and managers can communicate	

STRUCTURE	PROCESS	OUTCOME
Identified mechanisms are in place and known by department staff, i.e.	Nurses in management:	An informed workforce
team brief	provide clarity on the service mission and objectives	Involvement in decisions
regular newsletter		Supportive of ideas from staff
staff meetings	create a consultative approach to decision making	
Health Board/Trust plans and strategic information are accessible to managers		Honesty is valued
	ensure that written and verbal communications reach the identified people	Proactive, positive approach
Structured.formalised channels of communication exist	act as a 'syphon' for information	Staff have a sense of belonging
	provide staff within their responsibility with the necessary information to be effective	Staff have a corporate identity
Trusting, honest climate is created	develop feedback mechanisms and acknowledge time limits	
	monitor the effectiveness of existing communication systems	

Figure 2.6.6 *Standard for Management of Care*

Topic/Sub-Topic	Professional Accountability/Effective Management of Care	**Review Standard by Signature of CANO**
Client Group	Nursing Staff	
Ref	Nurses in Management	**Date**
Standard Statement	Nursing care is delivered and managed to provide continuity and excellence in practice	
Rationale	Necessary conditions and processes need to exist to facilitate practice which is dynamic, sensitive, relevant and responsive to patients	

STRUCTURE	PROCESS	OUTCOME
The head of each nursing care team: is a registered nurse with appropriate qualifications and recognised expertise in that clinical area is fully knowledgeable of budget allocation Health Board guidelines for nurse staffing establishments and grade mix or equivalent are available as a reference Organisation of nursing services is in place a) to provide continuity b) to facilitate nursing practice and the practice and implementation of nursing research Skills in selection/recruitment/retention of staff Clinical nurse specialist posts exist Formal links exist with in-service training and post basic education to facilitate learning A quality assurance programme exists which is compatible with the overall quality assurance strategy	The head of each nursing care team: negotiates with the nurse manager, the composition, in terms of skill mix of that team and the appointment of individuals ensures that nursing is developed systematically according to an agreed philosophy and model of care actively engages the team in setting, monitoring and evaluating standards of care is involved in succession planning Nurses are allocated to patients in a way that makes explicit the accountability for each patient's care from admission to discharge as well as on a daily basis The nurse accountable for the care of each patient acts on the patient's behalf and co-ordinates the patient's care	Each manager at this level: manages the team to ensure that the care is planned with each client, family and other professionals ensures that it is delivered to a professionally recognised standard ensures that it is evaluated to ensure effectiveness and quality ensures that development of the 'named nurse' is evident

Figure 2.6.7 *Standard for Quality Assurance Programme*

Topic/Sub-Topic	Management/Quality Assurance Programmes
Client Group	Nursing Staff
Ref	Nurses in Management
Standard Statement	Effective programmes exist for quality assurance and evaluation
Rationale	The development of quality assurance programmes in health care is a key aspect of management
Review Standard by	
Signature of CANO	
Date	

STRUCTURE	PROCESS	OUTCOME
A quality assurance programme exists which is compatible with the overall quality assurance strategy	Nurses in management:	Mechanisms identify shortcomings and enable action
Information on quality assurance is available	provide the agreed resources to execute the quality assurance programme and agreed changes	Mechanisms identify areas of good practice and enable the sharing of such practices
Local facilitator support exists	ensure criteria are set by which the manager can determine whether the stated objectives are achieved	Objectives are met within time limits
Staff have easy access to standards index	include the views of clients in the programme	Interprofessional collaboration is evident
Health Board and local strategy for quality assurance is available to staff	ensure that the quality assurance programme contains mechanisms for formulating criteria, agreeing standards, assessing the level of compliance, formulating action plans for the achievement of standards not being met	
Customers are aware of the quality assurance programme	ensure that the quality assurance programme identifies the quality assurance activities undertaken with other staff groups	
	take into account the amount of time spent on quality assurance activities when planning manpower levels	
	formulate action plans following the identification of any problems	
	regularly review the action plans with key personnel within predetermined time limits	

Figure 2.6.8 *Standard for Staff Interview Process*

Topic/Sub-Topic	Personnel/Staff Recruitment and Selection – The Interview Process	**Review Standard by**
Client Group	Interviewees	**Signature of CANO**
Ref	Personnel Services, Acute Unit	**Date**
Adopted by/Adapted by	Nurses in Management	
Standard Statement	The interview process is effective as a means of identifying the individual who most closely matches the requirements of the post and interview candidates are treated courteously and fairly	
Rationale	Selection of staff should be carried out in a fair and consistent manner which is a positive learning experience for both successful and unsuccessful interviewees	

STRUCTURE	PROCESS	OUTCOME
Environment A suitable waiting area is provided for the candidates	**Interview Structure** The appointing manager determines the structure and content of the interview and ensures that the approach is applied consistently to all candidates	Candidates are treated with courtesy and fairness at all times
The interview room is private and free from interruptions (including telephones/bleeps)	The panel members agree the areas of questioning bearing in mind the selection criteria	The interview process is effective as a means of identifying the individual who most closely matches the requirements of the post
The seating arrangements should reflect the style of the interview (i.e. formal or informal)	**Conducting the interview** The applicant is made to feel at ease	Unsuccessful candidates receive prompt and honest feedback on the reason for the decision and their performance at interview by either the appointing manager or personnel as appropriate
Documentation Information on candidates is treated in confidence and restricted to those members of staff involved directly in the recruitment process.	Appropriate background information is given on the unit and the post	All internal candidates are counselled regarding their applications by the appointing manager
Copies of application forms and job descriptions are made available to the panel members prior to the interviews	Initially questions are related to subjects familiar to the applicant	
	Questions which could be construed as discriminatory are avoided (e.g. sex, race, marital status, parental status)	

Figure 2.6.8 contd. *Standard for Staff Interview Process*

Topic/Sub-Topic	Personnel/Staff Recruitment and Selection – The Interview Process	**Review Standard by**
Client Group	Interviewees	**Signature of CANO**
Ref	Personnel Services, Acute Unit	**Date**
Adopted by/Adapted by	Nurses in Management	
Standard Statement	The interview process is effective as a means of identifying the individual who most closely matches the requirements of the post and interview candidates are treated courteously and fairly	
Rationale	Selection of staff should be carried out in a fair and consistent manner which is a positive learning experience for both successful and unsuccessful interviewees	

STRUCTURE	PROCESS	OUTCOME
Referers' reports and details of terms and conditions of service are made available to the appointing manager by personnel staff, providing two weeks' notice has been given of the shortlisted candidates	Applicants are informed of the terms and conditions of employment and health screening requirements	
	Applicants are given the chance to ask further questions at the end of the interview	
Membership of Panel	Where appropriate, registration details are checked	
The appointing manager determines membership of the panel which should be restricted to as few people as possible, all of whom should have a direct and legitimate interest in the appointment	Applicants are told when to expect the outcome of the interview and that unsuccessful applicants will be given the opportunity to discuss their interview	
	Following Interview	
	Immediately after the interview, notes will be written up reflecting the views of the panel	
	The appointing manager informs candidates verbally as to the outcome of the interview within the timescale laid down in unit recruitment procedures	

> "The heart of quality is not technique. It is a commitment by management to its people and product – stretching over a period of decades and lived with persistence and passion – that is unknown in most organizations today."
> (P Austin 1985, p118)
> A Passion for Excellence: The Leadership Difference, Warner Books, New York.

Index